Sustainable Development Goals Series

The **Sustainable Development Goals Series** is Springer Nature's inaugural cross-imprint book series that addresses and supports the United Nations' seventeen Sustainable Development Goals. The series fosters comprehensive research focused on these global targets and endeavours to address some of society's greatest grand challenges. The SDGs are inherently multidisciplinary, and they bring people working across different fields together and working towards a common goal. In this spirit, the Sustainable Development Goals series is the first at Springer Nature to publish books under both the Springer and Palgrave Macmillan imprints, bringing the strengths of our imprints together.

The Sustainable Development Goals Series is organized into eighteen subscries: one subseries based around each of the seventeen respective Sustainable Development Goals, and an eighteenth subseries, "Connecting the Goals," which serves as a home for volumes addressing multiple goals or studying the SDGs as a whole. Each subseries is guided by an expert Subseries Advisor with years or decades of experience studying and addressing core components of their respective Goal.

The SDG Series has a remit as broad as the SDGs themselves, and contributions are welcome from scientists, academics, policymakers, and researchers working in fields related to any of the seventeen goals. If you are interested in contributing a monograph or curated volume to the series, please contact the Publishers: Zachary Romano [Springer; zachary.romano@springer.com] and Rachael Ballard [Palgrave Macmillan; rachael.ballard@palgrave.com].

More information about this series at https://link.springer.com/bookseries/15486

Uta Schmidt-Straßburger

Editor

Improving Oncology Worldwide

Education, Clinical Research
and Global Cancer Care

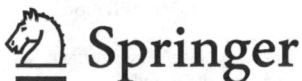 Springer

Editor
Uta Schmidt-Straßburger
Medical Faculty
University of Ulm
Ulm, Germany

ISSN 2523-3084   ISSN 2523-3092   (electronic)
Sustainable Development Goals Series
ISBN 978-3-030-96055-1   ISBN 978-3-030-96053-7   (eBook)
https://doi.org/10.1007/978-3-030-96053-7

To our patients and students, who instill in us the desire to be better professionals.
To our colleagues, who fight the same fights.
To our families, who support us in our pursuit to fight cancer and who take care of us when we come home bruised and battered.

Preface

Dear Reader,

When planning a meeting 2 years ago, a possible pandemic never even crossed my mind even though I was aware of the possibility, having read *The Coming Plague* by Laurie Garrett almost 25 years ago and having had to cancel the attendance of the Annual Meeting of the American Association for Cancer Research in Toronto in 2003. But life is full of surprises, good ones and the ones we strive to forget but that will still keep us up at night.

As the Scientific Director of the Advanced Oncology study program of Ulm University, my goal was to organize a riveting alumni meeting of previous and current students of our study program and to learn the progress they made in their areas of expertise at the Reisensburg Castle, a scientific retreat location belonging to Ulm University and the place for good networking.

Ensuring the smooth running of the study program is my primary occupation. I do that by ensuring its high quality and making contacts with highly qualified lecturers and supporting the students so they manage their studies successfully. However, I consider it also my duty to ensure that their studies give them the tools to thrive in their fight against cancer. This is what many of our current and past students set out to do in their own environments. Each one of us has made an impact in the lives of others. There might be roadblocks along the way, sometimes bumpers, sometimes huge obstacles like uprisings and wars. But we will always care for the people falling ill with cancers and make their lives better or at least more bearable.

Over the years, I have learned many things from my students, most of all resilience and perseverance. This is what this book is about: to make things better by bettering the education, by conducting research, and providing the best cancer care everywhere. This marathon is broken up into manageable pieces that you hopefully find inspiring to assess your own situation and apply knowledge there. Please feel free to reach out to the different authors—each one of them has put their heart into their chapter.

The selection of the authors was made based on their availability and my perception of their strength. Some of the authors I had requested had agreed at first and retracted later. The pandemic had its grip on them, making us miss the parts from Canada, or wars, which made the contributions from Libya and Iraq missing.

This book in its entirety shall contribute to the Sustainable Development Goal 3of the United Nations: "Ensure healthy lives and promote well-being for all at all ages." I think that the approaches described herein particularly aim at the defined targets 3.4, 3.8, 3b, and 3c.

The alumni meeting, which this book is based upon, was held virtually in October 2020. It was sad to not be able to meet in person, but then, the upside was that so many more people could attend and be inspired. The comradery was our usual one, and we were happy to learn from each other. I hope, you will be, too.

Ulm, Germany   Uta Schmidt-Straßburger
June 2021

Acknowledgments

People

Thank you to all the authors and discussants for your contributions during the meeting and for writing your chapters. We made it!

This book would not be possible without the support of our infrastructure, the Advanced Oncology core team and its present members, Ms. Bettina Wabitsch, Ms. Ursula Russo, and Mr. Sebastian Dannenberg, and the Division of Learning and Teaching, particularly its head, Dr. Claudia Grab-Kroll, but also all the other lovely people involved in e-education and educational research.

The Comprehensive Cancer Center Ulm has supported the study program right from the beginning, through the years and continues to do so. I am particularly grateful to Prof. Hartmut Döhner, Prof. Thomas Seufferlein and Prof. Stephan Stilgenbauer for their unwavering support and contributions. I am at least equally indebted to Ms. Colette Meister for her work, insight, and help.

A big thank you to the administrators of the German Academic Exchange Service (Deutscher Akademischer Austauschdienst, DAAD), Ms. Leokadia Staffa and Ms. Arngard Leifert, for being at my disposal whenever I had a question.

I want to thank the people of Springer Nature for guiding me through the publishing process, particularly Ms. Antonella Cerri and Ms. Niveka Somasundaram.

Funding Body

The funds for publishing this book were attributed to the study program by the DAAD.

About the Book

Improving Oncology Worldwide is unique in that it describes strategies and experiences of highly skilled professionals in improving oncology care worldwide. The contributors have studied at Ulm University in the past and have had exposure to the ESMO/ASCO global curriculum in oncology or are part of Ulm University faculty.

The book is structured into three parts with several chapters each, reflecting the individual experiences. It covers ways to improve oncology education and scientific training, how do we set up and run a clinical research facility ethically and efficiently, but mostly it addresses the challenges that the workforce encounters in the real world. It addresses real-world oncologists all over the world and their allies throughout the associated industries.

One possible solution to meet the growing demand in oncology *education* is to provide e-learning or blended learning. Science education and good scientific practice are other aspects. How to set up medical training in a low- or middle-income setting so that all parties will be satisfied with the outcome?

Clinical research in the field of oncology is currently in full bloom due to the coming of age of targeted therapies as well as the advent of immune therapy. Experiences in setting up relevant infrastructures in low- and middle-income settings are being shared as well as the experiences from the "other" side, high-income settings, and the pharmaceutical industry. The contributions strive to demonstrate how to perform good science in low- and middle-income settings.

The main challenge remains the daily patient care of the oncologist. Needs differ for patients and physicians depending on the factors like peace, social and gender equality. The main challenges of today's oncologists seem to be the ever-growing *patient care* and administrative workload and the risk of burn-out. What are the best strategies to maintain a healthy work-life for the benefit of the patients, the physicians, and society?

Based on single contributions by alumni and faculty of the study program, the three parts contain summarizing articles. The authors of these chapters bring the single contributions to the next level by drawing conclusions about the projects presented and the ensuing discussions among the participants of the meeting. In other words, even though the different contributions will be aimed at particular targets of the presenter's own experience, the main aim of this entire book is to draw conclusions that are valid beyond the setting of an alumni workshop and that line out areas of need for further improvement in addition to the solutions introduced already.

Contents

Contributors

Patriciu-Andrei Achimaş-Cadariu Iuliu Hatieganu University of Medicine and Pharmacy, Cluj-Napoca, Romania

Ion Chiricuta Institute of Oncology, Cluj-Napoca, Romania

Ahmad Samir Alfaar Experimental Ophthalmology, Charité—Universitätsmedizin Berlin, Berlin, Berlin, Germany

Department of Ophthalmology, University Hospital of Giessen and Marburg, Giessen, Germany

Carlos A. Castaneda Department of Medical Oncology, Instituto Nacional de Enfermedades Neoplásicas, Lima, Peru

Zeinab Elsayed Clinical Oncology Department, Ain Shams University Hospitals, Abbassia, Cairo, Egypt

Bruno Lemos Ferrari Department of Medical Oncology, Oncocentro de Minas Gerais, Belo Horizonte, Minas Gerais, Brazil

Oncoclinicas Group, São Paulo, SP, Brazil

Andre A. J. Gemeinder de Moraes Clinical Research Unity, Centro de Oncologia Campinas, Campinas, SP, Brazil

Rodrigo Cunha Guimaraes Department of Medical Oncology, Oncocentro de Minas Gerais, Belo Horizonte, Minas Gerais, Brazil

Ninad Katdare Department of Surgical Oncology, HCG Cancer Centre, Mumbai, Maharashtra, India

Mohamed Reda Kelany Clinical Oncology Department, Ain Shams University Hospitals, Abbassia, Cairo, Egypt

Nicole Lang Medical Faculty and University Hospital of Ulm, Ulm, Germany

Layth Mula-Hussain Radiation Oncology, College of Medicine—Ninevah University, Mosul, Iraq

Atara Ntekim Department of Radiation Oncology, College of Medicine, University of Ibadan Nigeria, Ibadan, Nigeria

Judy Vicente de Paulo Portuguese Insitute of Oncology of Coimbra, Coimbra, Portugal

Mirosława Püsküllüoğlu Department of Clinical Oncology, Maria Sklodowska-Curie National Research Institute of Oncology, Krakow, Poland

Faculty of Medicine, Department of Medical Education, Jagiellonian University Medical College, Krakow, Poland

Ahmed Magdy Rabea Medical Oncology Department, Shefa El Orman Hospital, Luxor, Egypt

Medical Oncology Department, National Cancer Institute, Cairo University, Cairo, Egypt

Amir Radfar Medical Education, University of Central Florida, Orlando, FL, USA

Blanca Iciar Indave Ruiz WHO Classification of Tumours Group, International Agency for Research on Cancer, Lyon, France

Pedro Ribeiro Santos Department of Medical Oncology, Oncocentro de Minas Gerais, Belo Horizonte, Minas Gerais, Brazil

Uta Schmidt-Straßburger Advanced Oncology Study Program, Division of Learning and Teaching, Deanery of the Medical Faculty, Ulm, Germany

Thomas Seufferlein Department of Internal Medicine I, Ulm University Hospital and Ulm Comprehensive Cancer Center CCCU, Ulm, Germany

Velizar Shivarov Faculty of Biology, Department of Genetics, St. Kliment Ohridski Sofia University, Sofia, Bulgaria

PRAHS, Sofia, Bulgaria

Gevorg Tamamyan Pediatric Cancer and Blood Disorders Center of Armenia, Hematology Center After Prof. R.H. Yeolyan, Yerevan, Armenia

Department of Pediatric Oncology and Hematology, Yerevan State Medical University, Yerevan, Armenia

Master Program in Advanced Oncology, University of Ulm, Ulm, Germany

Abbreviations

AACR	American Association for Cancer Research
ASCO	American Society of Clinical Oncology
ASTRO	American Society for Radiation Oncology
b-learning	Blended learning, a mixture of e-learning and learning in attendance
COVID-19	Coronavirus disease 2019
ECTS	European Credit Transfer and Accumulation System
edX	An American massive open online course provider
e-learning	Learning using online resources
ESMO	European Society for Medical Oncology
ESO	European School of Oncology
ESTRO	European Society for Radiotherapy and Oncology
GCP	Good Clinical Practice
HIC	High-Income Country
IARC	International Agency for Research on Cancer
LMIC	Low- and Middle-Income Countries
MOOC	Massive Open Online Course
NCCP	National Cancer Control Plan
NCI	National Cancer Institute
Sars-CoV-2	Severe acute respiratory syndrome coronavirus 2
SPOC	Small Private Online Course
UICC	Union for International Cancer Control
WCT	WHO Classification of Tumours group
WHO	World Health Organization

Part I
Education

Improving Education: A Global Perspective

Mirosława Püsküllüoğlu

The Challenges in Oncology Education

Continuing medical education (CME) is an important topic in current medical practice including the oncology field. The discussion about how to implement CME in oncologists' training is not a novelty and has been taking place during the last few decades (Emiliani 1998). Building structured pathways in under- and post-graduate medical training allows proper quality of offered programs or educational events and assures equal chances in knowledge and skills gaining. However, harmonization in oncologists' training meets obstacles that result from significant differences in specialization trainings (e.g., length of training, duration of initial training in internal medicine) and distribution of patients between different specialists that may vary from country to country. Taking into consideration Europe, we may see the local discrepancies. In most countries, medical oncology is recognized as a separate specialty (e.g., Spain, Romania, or Switzerland); in others, it is a subspecialty (e.g., Turkey) and is mixed with hematology (e.g., Germany) or radiotherapy (e.g., Sweden). There are still some countries where there is no official training in this specialty (Pavlidis et al. 2016). The situation for the training in radiation oncology is even more complicated. For example, Poland offers specialization in clinical oncology and radiotherapy. Clinical oncologists are de facto trained five and a half years to work as medical oncologists with 2 years of initial internal medicine involvement, and radiotherapists are trained to provide radiation therapy while they are commonly responsible for systemic treatment during radiochemotherapy. Thus, there is also a matter of local nomenclature.

The challenges in oncology education both locally and globally, especially in the postgraduate area, can be divided into (I) general issues common for all medical fields such as the following:

- Limited guidelines provided by international societies in the area of medical education.
- Lack of training/residency program harmonization.
- Differences between countries in the access to local and international training activities (e.g., due to financial issues).
- Differences between countries in the access (as a trainee) to top reference cancer care centers.

M. Püsküllüoğlu (✉)
Department of Clinical Oncology, Maria Sklodowska-Curie National Research Institute of Oncology, Krakow, Poland

Faculty of Medicine, Department of Medical Education, Jagiellonian University Medical College, Krakow, Poland

© The Author(s) 2022
U. Schmidt-Strassburger (ed.), *Improving Oncology Worldwide*, Sustainable Development Goals Series, https://doi.org/10.1007/978-3-030-96053-7_1

- Differences between countries in legal regulations or access to electronic and blended learning (e- and b-learning) activities.
- Challenges with obtaining a networking experience.
- Challenges with direct transfer of know-how from higher to lower developed countries.
- Lack of qualified medical staff in many parts of the world (trainers/faculty members).
- Lack of medical education training activities provided for trainers/faculty members.

Challenges can also be divided into (II) area specific for oncology such as the following:

- Differences between countries in the reimbursement process or access to new oncology drugs (thus, difficulties in obtaining practical experience).
- Lack of harmonization in patient pathways/area of expertise of different experts (e.g., systemic treatment of skin malignancies can be a subject of interest of dermatologists or medical oncologists depending on country).
- Major differences in training pathways for clinical oncologists, medical oncologists, and radiotherapists between countries.

The European Society for Medical Oncology (ESMO)/American Society of Clinical Oncology (ASCO) global curriculum in oncology provides detailed international guidelines for oncology training (Hansen et al. 2004; Dittrich et al. 2016). Following this strategy can result in harmonization of postgraduate oncology education all over the world. Unfortunately, any attempt of introducing these guidelines in different countries might meet obstacles resulting from financial or cultural discrepancies, particularly when transferring the guidelines to low- and middle-income countries (LMICs) but not limited to these settings.

Some examples of these challenges can be shifting the training from theoretical to practical, introducing research activities, overcoming the resistance from the faculty resulting from their work overload and lack of being paid for educational supervision, the trainees' resistance that can be connected to their fear of new assessment methods introduced, and possible retaliation by superiors when being too frank in the assessment of a training program.

Using an e-learning or b-learning (blended learning) approach in medical education is not a novelty anymore. This approach has its well-known advantages but also numerous challenges, for example, choosing proper evaluation methods (O'Doherty et al. 2018; de Leeuw et al. 2019). A great example in oncology is an international blended learning program introduced by the University of Ulm more than a decade ago. More and more good quality offers are being introduced into the market with an example of an e-learning program regarding the use of evidence-based approach in improving World Health Organization (WHO) Classification of Tumours books. With introducing e-programs (as MOOCs, Massive Open Online Courses; or SPOCs, Small Private Online Courses discussed later), there is always a hope of facilitating the participation of oncologists from LMICs and a question about advertising such activity among them. Such educational activities can support building proper personal networking also among oncologists from LMICs allowing them easy access to international know-how but also enabling sharing their practical knowledge in running oncology centers and building educational structures with more limited financial support. Knowing their experience can help the others to define potential complications and to build a strategy for overcoming these obstacles. Scientific societies may offer smaller didactic bites, but uptake by professionals has been slow and with only very little adherence. This raises the question again on how to successfully implement the curricula described.

While focusing on harmonization of global oncology training or introducing new technologies into cancer education, one cannot forget that in many regions of the world, the lack of qualified personnel and facilities and general poverty require to do a step back and make more basic efforts to build an oncology training program from scratch. Setting up medical training in LMICs is an especially demanding task, and the results cannot be expected quickly. During the past 15 years, we have observed a general decay in global stability paired with considerable human capital flight from regions of war, hunger, and any other instability. Wealthier countries profit from this exodus of highly skilled manpower, but the regions left behind experience an increasing drought of well-qualified personnel and henceforth a widening gap in healthcare provision.

2020 being a year of SARS-CoV-2 brought additional problems in patients' care and medical education in oncology. Cancer patients were exposed to a delay in diagnostic and treatment procedures, but also oncologists, being involved in restructuring of treatment forces, lost numerous opportunities of in-person training programs or continuing planned specialization trainings. However, one cannot say this year was "lost for oncology education development." Switching numerous top activities from in-class to e-meetings allowed the contribution and active participation of a greater number of participants. What is more, paradoxically, initially it was helpful in reducing the discrepancy between countries in the access to good quality activities in oncology but also accelerated the decision of introducing e-activities into obligatory oncology training in numerous countries. 2021 being a year of vaccination has already shown a great discrepancy in the access to SARS-CoV-2 vaccines between high- and low-income countries. It is likely to contribute to a further deepening of medical education inequality.

Improving Education in Oncology: Real-Life Examples

Uta Schmidt-Straßburger, a scientific director of the Advanced Oncology Study Programme at the University of Ulm, presents a summary of a 10-year experience in continuous development and improvement of b-learning program created for oncologists and their colleagues. By implementing ESMO/ASCO recommendations for a global curriculum in oncology and organizing the material into seven modules, the program assured standardization and comprehensiveness. Adding soft skills workshops, for example, in negotiation or presentation, and assuring personal coaching and international environment created a unique opportunity for participants to build a very strong and supportive network. Probably the biggest potential in the studies lies in the strong interpersonal interactions among participants, staff, and associated researchers and tutors that have already resulted in numerous projects and led to further development of former students even after the graduation from the program. Such a network plays a role not only in exchanging opinions, experience, and views but also is a solid ground for building didactic, scientific, translational, and clinical projects.

Similar to the master classes in clinical oncology organized by the European School of Oncology (ESO) together with ESMO, the personal interactions between participants, organizers, and faculty create long-lasting positive associations with a lifelong learning experience in oncology and encourage participants to join networks of continuing medical education like e-ESO and to convene at ESMO annual meetings.

A good example on how to build the local curriculum for oncologists basing on the ESMO/ASCO recommendations can be provided by Zeinab Elsayed and Mohamed Reda Kelany—oncologists working in Egypt. The transfer of know-how cannot be direct in such situations as the socioeconomic and cultural background since, for example, former specialist training requirements, accreditation and organization of oncology centers, and the financing system are completely different. Some of the obstacles are common for a majority of countries, whereas others are cultural and financially dependent. Factors such as the risk of burnout or difficulties in motivating the busy faculty staff to devote the time to residents' training are more general, and oncologists all over the world face these problems. On the other hand, limited facilities, shorter duration of a specialty training, and lack of research options are more specific for LMICs (Murali and Banerjee 2018; Burki 2018; Jalan et al. 2020).

Ahmed Magdy Rabea shares some practical solutions that were introduced in one of the oncology centers in Luxor. He managed to transfer and propagate well-known solutions such as regular educational lectures, clinical pharmacists' meetings, and daily clinical rounds for residents and fellows. Supporting international training of the residents can bring future benefits to the parent unit, but one needs to be aware that it means loss on manpower at the beginning of such investment.

Building from scratch a national network for sarcoma treatment in Egypt seems extremely challenging. Mohamed Reda Kelany presents strengths, weaknesses, opportunities, and threats of the proposed sarcoma network. It is highlighted that even such project created from scratch needs patient advocate groups and the stakeholders representing different discipline involvements so as to make the effort lasting and sustainable.

The number of obstacles to face with and a massive effort while building an oncology educational program from the beginning is presented by Layth Mula-Hussain, a lecturer in radiation oncology from Iraq. The first board-certified residency program in radiation oncology was launched between 2013 and 2017 in Iraq (Mula-Hussain et al. 2019). Sharing this experience is extremely valuable as the problem was defined not only in the lacking procedures but also lack of staff or facilities. It is not an exaggeration to say that the presented example addressed almost all the challenges of postgraduate medical education, both general and specific for oncology, those present all over the world, and characteristic for LMICs. Four years after the program's establishment, its authors can pass the updated knowledge and know-how to other colleagues. Ten physicians completed the training in radiation oncology between 2017 and 2020 allowing the care for the population of over ten million people. When trying to find the main factors responsible for this success, two facts cannot be neglected: the preparation period was long including technical and logistical planning and the faculty setup to create the syllabus consisted of local and external specialists. That would not

be possible without the preexisting network organization.

How to set up a new program is also a topic for Blanca Iciar Indave Ruiz, a research assistant currently working at the International Agency for Research on Cancer and World Health Organization (WHO) Classification of Tumours Group. However, this time the goal is to build an online training program named Evi-Pat and propagate high-quality and well-functioning scientific activities, that is, further work on the WHO Classification of Tumours by an evidence-based approach in order to improve adopting these methods. The main educational obstacles in this situation are more specific for e- and b-learning. Apart from obvious ones, choosing the proper virtual learning environment (VLE) or evaluation methodology, new challenges appeared, for example, how to advertise internationally, how to define and reach proper course recipients, and how to obtain additional funding to build such a program. To deal with potential issues, a collaboration between partners was established: the Master Online Advanced Oncology program at the University of Ulm, the Cochrane Netherlands, the Universidade Estadual de Campinas in Brazil, and the WHO Classification of Tumours. This is a new initiative, where in order to keep the reliability of tumor classification, addressing critical questions and finding research gaps seem crucial.

The presented list of real-life examples is not limited to transferring knowledge from high- to low-income countries or supporting to build other successful online programs. A great model of how the activities of current and former students and staff can serve also in high-income country is presented by Judy Vicente de Paulo, a medical oncologist from Portugal and a president of the Young Oncologists Committee of the Portuguese Society of Oncology in a section: Continuing education for the young oncology workforce in Portugal. These initiatives are frequent in developed countries where oncologists in training take over partial responsibility for their training and its improvement with a support from ESMO or national societies. The Nucleus of Interns and Young Specialists of the Portuguese Society of Oncology was founded in 2015. The chapter summarizes the challenges that young oncologists face during the residency program in Portugal and the solutions implemented to meet these challenges including soft skills workshops or additional training to cover hot topics in oncology like oncological emergencies. Currently, a similar initiative has been born in Poland.

Conclusions

This section summarized the exemplary projects run by participants and supervisors engaged in the Master Online Advanced Oncology program at the University of Ulm—researchers and physicians representing various fields of oncology, living in different parts of the world, facing challenges typical for countries with high, middle, and low income, and representing all steps of career pathway from residents in training to chairs of departments. It is worth noticing that while debating on these projects, all challenges in oncology education pointed out at the beginning of this chapter were covered.

References

Burki TK (2018) Oncologists burnout in the spotlight. Lancet Oncol 19(5):e238

de Leeuw R, de Soet A, van der Horst S, Walsh K, Westerman M, Scheele F (2019) How we evaluate postgraduate medical E-learning: systematic review. JMIR Med Educ 5(1):e13128

Dittrich C, Kosty M, Jezdic S, Pyle D, Berardi R, Bergh J et al (2016) ESMO/ASCO recommendations for a global curriculum in medical oncology edition 2016. Open 1:97. http://esmoopen.bmj.com/

Emiliani E (1998) Continuing medical education in radiation oncology. Tumori 84(2):96–100

Hansen HH, Bajorin DF, Muss HB, Purkalne G, Schrijvers D, Stahel R (2004) Recommendations for a Global Core Curriculum in Medical Oncology Special article Recommendations for a Global Core Curriculum in Medical Oncology ESMO/ASCO Task Force on Global Curriculum in Medical Oncology [cited 2021 May 31]; www.zora.uzh.churl. https://doi.org/10.5167/uzh-155120

Jalan D, Rubagumya F, Hopman WM, Vanderpuye V, Lopes G, Seruga B et al (2020) Training of oncologists: results of a global survey. Ecancermedicalscience 14:1074

Mula-Hussain L, Shamsaldin AN, Al-Ghazi M, Muhammad HA, Wadi-Ramahi S, Hanna RK et al (2019) Board-certified specialty training program in radiation oncology in a war-torn country: challenges, solutions and outcomes. Clin Transl Radiat Oncol 19:46–51. https://www.sciencedirect.com/science/article/pii/S2405630819300904

Murali K, Banerjee S (2018) Burnout in oncologists is a serious issue: what can we do about it? Cancer Treat Rev 68:55–61

Pavlidis N, Alba E, Berardi R, Bergh J, El Saghir N, Jassem J et al (2016) The ESMO/ASCO global curriculum and the evolution of medical oncology training in Europe. ESMO Open 1(1):e000004

O'Doherty D, Dromey M, Lougheed J, Hannigan A, Last J, McGrath D (2018) Barriers and solutions to online learning in medical education – an integrative review. BMC Med Educ 18(1):130

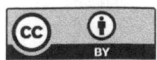

Blended Learning for Oncologists and Their Colleagues

Uta Schmidt-Straßburger

ESMO/ASCO Recommendations for a Global Curriculum in Medical Oncology

The first recommendations for a global curriculum in medical oncology were published and distributed worldwide by a joint taskforce of the European Society for Medical Oncology (ESMO) and the American Society of Clinical Oncology (ASCO) in 2004 (Hansen et al. 2004). These recommendations were comprehensively updated in 2010 and 2016 (Dittrich et al. 2016). Their currently available form has been endorsed by 51 different professional organizations linked to oncology and translated into 8 languages different from English thereby making it accessible to professionals throughout the world (ESMO 2021).

From the start, the recommendations covered all aspects of oncology training such as the structural prerequisites of a proper training program, the contents, and the skillset that trainees should strive to achieve. The most recent edition of the curriculum was supplemented with an extensive logbook detailing the required procedures (ESMO 2021). On 240 pages, items are categorized according to the respective area, entity, or essential procedure, and a before/after assessment is done by the direct supervisor/mentor. The assessment is to be countersigned by the trainee and the head/director of the respective department or clinic. Many specialists from both scientific societies, ESMO and ASCO, have contributed to this very fine-grained curriculum and created a blueprint for entire generations of oncologists. I cannot emphasize enough the outreach effect of this curriculum on specialists all over the world.

A very important innovation was introduced into the third edition in 2016: the level of competence (ESMO 2021). Three different levels of competence have been defined: awareness, knowledge, and skill. While it is easy to be aware of a fact, a concept, or a procedure, it is an entirely different level to really know or even master them. How can a new level of competence be reached? Of course, clinical training should teach the skills to competently treat cancer patients and provide not only medication but also any support that the patient or their family might need. But it must be accompanied by didactic training to explain and internalize the concepts of the underlying biology, accompanying diagnostics, treatment plans, entity-specific issues, as well as training for professional communication with patients, peers, and other stakeholders in the cancer care continuum.

U. Schmidt-Straßburger (✉)
Advanced Oncology Study Program, Division of Learning and Teaching, Deanery of the Medical Faculty, Ulm, Germany
e-mail: uta.schmidt-strassburger@uni-ulm.de

U. Schmidt-Strassburger (ed.), *Improving Oncology Worldwide*, Sustainable Development Goals Series, https://doi.org/10.1007/978-3-030-96053-7_2

Of MOOCs (Massive Open Online Courses) and SPOCs (Small Private Online Courses)

Both ESMO and ASCO are providing didactical online material on a pay per service rate at their websites so that interested professionals can assess the videos and quizzes in order to learn points outlined in the global curriculum. There are discounts available for learners in training as well as for learners from low- and middle-income countries (LMICs). As with professional life in general, these teaching materials are available in an asynchronous manner, that is, learners may access them depending on their schedules and preferences. Herein lies also a major hindrance in the use of these materials: learning is self-paced and enforced by board certification or maintenance of certification examinations (Yuan and Powell 2015). An explorative analysis by ASCO showed that the group of learning professionals is highly heterogeneous in terms of learners' preferences (George et al. 2021). Many professional societies require a documentation of continuous medical education as part of ongoing licensure. These activities may comprise in-person events like meetings and courses and electronic activities like quizzes and didactic videos. There are country-specific differences in the requirements for admissions to certification examinations or maintenance of certification making offered online materials by ESMO or ASCO less palatable to physicians outside of the scientific society's country/region.

What can be done to offer a comprehensive didactic education in oncology? The conventional route would probably be to establish a dedicated structured PhD program for oncologists and provide the necessary didactic teaching. Another option would be to guide trainees and other interested professionals didactically in a more decentralized manner but guide them nonetheless. The question is as follows: by what didactic approach and with what level of supervision?

With the coming of age of information technology (IT) and the Internet, possibilities to share knowledge have grown exponentially. The openness of the Internet led also to attempts of making education more equitable, at least to the outside viewer (Yuan and Powell 2013). One of the results was the generation of MOOCs (massive open online courses). These courses contain didactical material and address learners' needs in terms of contents. Frequently, they are offered by established high-ranking universities building on successful in-person courses or serving as both an outreach and a teaser, edX courses, for example. Many of these courses, either free of charge or available at affordable prices, had many subscribers to start with and rather little numbers of finishers owing to the fact that curricular obligations like assignments posed barriers for the learners involved in these courses. Another challenge is that the registration for MOOCs is done technically, and there is no person-to-person contact involved at first, likely to result in less identification with the goals and lower adherence. Many programs do involve group work and group assignments, though, and there is people-machine-machine-people interaction involved making the course curricula more adapted to the learners' needs for human communication. The general didactics of MOOCs are based on andragogy, just like every "normal" course one might follow in person at university. They are oftentimes even more learner-centered than a conventional lecture in a medium university like ours, with approximately 350 students in order to keep the learner engaged as long as possible.

SPOCs (small private online courses) are different. Being small brings a different level of engagement between course organizers and learners. The privacy is usually enabled by paying tuition to cover the costs of the entire endeavor, that is, the personnel for organizing and running the course, particularly tutors to engage and activate the learners. Many universities offer such courses, and some of them are not small at all. These courses very often are conducted in a setting that combines attendance in person with online learning phases and is therefore called blended.

At Ulm University, we have currently seven study programs that are built upon the blended learning concepts, and the Advanced Oncology study program was the first among these. Why was it established? What are the benefits for the learners? Is there a benefit for the university?

A Broader Vision

It started with a true pioneer in his field, Theodor Max Fliedner (TMF). He was trained in internal medicine, particularly hematology. Early on in his career, he investigated the effects of radiation on the bone marrow and continued to do so beyond his retirement. He was one of the pioneers of stem cell research within the context of leukemia. One of his inventions, the "Ulmer Zelt" (Life Island), is still being used in order to keep patients germ-free after bone marrow transplants (Hoelzer and Gale 2016). TMF was among the founders of Ulm University, was the university's president from 1983 until 1991, and worked afterward as a medical liaison for WHO by chairing the Global Advisory Committee on Health Research between 1993 and 1997 (Weber-Tuckermann 2016). In other words, he was at ease with the subcellular, cellular, organismal, and all organizational levels of cancer and cancer research.

As can be taken from his final report to WHO, things were clear to TMF from an epidemiological perspective: registries should be established to report incidence and mortality of cancer in a population. Then physicians must find, test, and apply new treatments to lower incidence and mortality. Their outcomes are measured by reporting to registries and benchmarking the data; comparing them with the previously reported ones; taking action depending on the outcome of the reporting, that is, being satisfied with the achievements or being dissatisfied with the achievements; and engaging into further iterations of the cycle (World Health Organization 1998), if only things were not muddied by the tiny little details!

In "the" agenda, TMF also described telehealth approaches and distance learning using the (French) term telematic (World Health Organization 1998). And this is actually what he focused on during the last years of his life, to lay the foundation for a network of oncologists, who want to further educate themselves to conquer cancer in their countries. Problems were challenges and to be solved and that was that. In project management, we often talk about stakeholders and ownership, and this was practiced by TMF by engaging in wider discussions about long-term goals or even visions. Those, who had worked with him, know that TMF ensured that his visions materialized.

The Ulm University Advanced Oncology Study Program

In 2008, Ulm University successfully applied for a grant for establishing its first blended learning program, Advanced Oncology. At the core of this degree-awarding study program are the four online modules "Interdisciplinary Oncology," "Clinical Research," "Advanced Therapies and Integrated Concepts," and "Management." These modules are embedded in a teaching concept that covers soft skills and knowledge but also networking activities.

Summer School "Challenges and Introduction"

During this—usually—in-person meeting, organizers and students meet for the very first time. Students are being welcomed and formally enrolled, that is, they present the original documents that were the basis for their admission to the study program. This is followed by the mutual introduction as well as the introduction to all issues pertaining to the organization of the study program including the Master's theses. The students learn the use of the Moodle-based learning platform, how to interact with the lecturers and each other, and how to take the mandatory pre-exam assignments that are required for the admission to the module examinations. This kickoff meeting is very inspirational, and we have optimized it over more than 10 years that we run the program. According to the students' wishes, introductory lectures by module responsibles were reduced in favor of more interactive aspects like the pathology catch-up and workshop as well as a first introduction of the health economic assessments. In order to accompany this professional growth, we also provide personal coaching throughout the time of studies if requested by the students. The coach introduces herself and her coaching method during this seminar. Starting in 2019, we welcomed a colleague of the WHO Classification of Tumours Group, who introduces students to evidence-based medicine and contributes to the workshop by teaching critical appraisal of published literature. The other topics of the workshop relate to molecular diagnostics and digital pathology. All this is then observed on a professional level during a visit of one of the tumor boards of the Comprehensive Cancer Center Ulm (CCCU), usually the leukemia and lymphoma board. Students return to their home countries, well-instructed and primed for the things to come.

Module "Interdisciplinary Oncology"

This module is divided into the courses "Cellular and Molecular Biology of Cancer," "Diagnostics," "Principles of Therapy and Treatment," and "Epidemiology."

The first course comprises a bouquet of lectures that address the underlying biology and biochemistry of cancer formation, evasion, and metastasis. Besides the obvious relation to the study subject, this course serves the didactical purpose to reactivate learning strategies of the students and to encourage them to ask the expert lecturers questions pertaining to the subject matter. All lecturers can provide knowledge and guidance beyond their lectures, and this is essential to overcome long existing reluctance to the matter at hand for most of the physicians studying with us. Scientists usually have less trouble following these lectures. This course, like all the subsequent ones, needs to be passed in order to be admitted to the module examination.

The course "Diagnostics" covers topics from histopathological assessment of specimens to whole-body imaging. Many aspects of the previous course like the molecular targets are automatically rehearsed since their diagnostic and/or prognostic value had been clinically proven. During the course "Principles of Therapy and Treatment," students familiarize themselves with all aspects of treating tumors or patients with tumors in general, starting from immunotherapy and ending with genetic counseling and stem cell transplantation. Lastly, our dedicated epidemiologist explains in detail cancer statistics, registries, and the resources offered by the International Agency for Research on Cancer (IARC) during the course "Epidemiology".

By the end of the winter term, students return to Ulm to take their first online examination; attend a workshop on molecular diagnostics, one on scientific writing; and start working toward the "Biometry" course of the upcoming module. Their favorite part, however, is an entire day of soft skill training with a professional communication trainer. Using direct feedback by peers supported by individually recorded videos, students polish their rhetoric strengths and are able to make a better first (and second) impression.

Module "Clinical Research"

This module covers the entire topic of good clinical practice (GCP), biometry, and project management together with ethical issues that may arise during the proper conduct of clinical research.

The course "Biometry" empowers the students to understand and properly handle numbers linked to anything that is measurable. Even though this course is feared by many students in the beginning, the overwhelmingly good results in the module examinations speak for themselves. "Clinical Trials" covers all aspects of clinical trials, starting from the concept of evidence generation, detailed descriptions of the different and particularly critical phases of clinical trials, and the transfer of study results into clinical practice. This is followed by the short, but very important, course "Ethical Aspects," detailing the legal and ethical obligations of researchers and how to prevent and detect scientific misconduct. Observational studies are introduced as well as the principles and proper conduct of systematic reviews and meta-analyses. Finally, students learn aspects of project management and biosimilars and rehearse health economic evaluations.

After a thorough in-person repetition of all things in "Biometry", students take their examinations and visit a production plant for biosimilars. The third seminar marks the point in time, when students have finished half of the curriculum. The students meet the elder class for the first time and network with them. Also, they refine their communication and negotiation skills and join the elder class, when those students present their thesis projects. In order to enable the students to write their own theses, aspects of scientific writing are covered in a workshop. At the end of the seminar, the younger class joins the elder one for the graduation ceremony of the elder class.

Module "Advanced Therapies and Integrated Concepts"

This module is composed of the courses on clinical oncology as well as one that covers entity-overarching aspects of cancer patient care.

The two courses on clinical oncology cover the epidemiology, etiology, diagnostics, and multidisciplinary therapy of breast and gynecological cancers, urogenital cancers, cancers of the gastrointestinal tract, lung cancers, head and neck cancers, sarcomas, melanoma, cancers of the nervous system, cancers of unknown primary, HIV-associated malignancies, and tumors of the hematopoietic and lymphoid tissues as well as pediatric tumors. This intense agenda is supplemented by the course "Integrated Therapeutic Concepts," which addresses palliative care, pain therapy, evidence-based complementary therapy, psycho-oncology, and communication and counseling.

The hard work on this module is compensated by the overwhelming experience of being part of the ESO (European Southern Observatory)/

ESMO master class in clinical oncology. Before joining this live event, our students take their module examination and follow the five-day immersion in clinical oncology with European leaders and many master class participants from other countries. An essential part of this master class has been the training in difficult communication scenarios with professional actors and the instructive feedback together with the individual case presentations by the master class participants. This event is also a good bonding experience for each one of the participating classes. The "Ulm group" is frequently perceived as an entity and less as individuals. For the students, this learning and socializing experience is another highlight of their studies.

Module "Management"

The last online module of this curriculum consists of the courses "Business Basics," "Health-Care System," "Management of Entities and Processes," and "Quality Control."

The first course introduces concepts of business administration to the health-care professionals. Apart from managerial concepts and financial aspects, modern concepts of good governance are introduced, focusing on the needs of our learners. Next, a comparative assessment of health-care systems lines out different aspects of health-care organization in different countries and their benefits and disadvantages for patients. Using the German social security system as an example, decision-making in this system and cash flows are highlighted. "Management of Entities and Processes" contains lectures on the overarching concepts of WHO's vision on cancer care, national cancer control plans (NCCPs), certification of tumor centers; management of practices, hospitals, and telemedicine; and ways on how to optimize clinical pathways. The course on quality control addresses individual points that need to be adjusted for proper quality control and improvement of cancer care including change management.

As usual, students take their module examination before exploring certain managerial aspects further. This comprises decision-making on the prices of cancer drugs, negotiation training, and a workshop on the optimization of clinical pathways. Being now the elder class, the students meet the younger class for the first time and network.

Summer School "Future Perspectives"

The second part of the last attendance seminar is the most exciting one because all students of the elder class present the status of their master's thesis projects to three different groups, their supervisors, their peers, and the younger class. These presentations take place at the Reisensburg castle, a scientific meeting venue of Ulm University. In an intense exchange, data and concepts are being discussed, and suggestions for improvement are being made by supervisors and students alike. Personally, I like this part of the last seminar best, because the science is the most appealing part to me, and I observe the growth each and every student made during the course of their studies. This is also the moment, where supervisors and students engage in conversations as peers—as one would expect from learners achieving the next step and mentors accepting their mentees in their circle. It is then that everyone in the class is supported by all the students not presenting, and it forms a moving personal experience of having grown as a group, as a person, as a scientist, and as an expert.

The younger class is oftentimes a little bit intimidated by flawless presentations of their elders. This helps to encourage the youngsters to pursue their own thesis projects dutifully and knowingly. Most of all, it helps to identify all people present whom to network with on certain aspects of patient care or basic research, and this is an inherent feature of this study program.

In line with this are the graduation on the evening of the joint thesis presentations and the seminar on future perspectives, where we reflect together on aspects of improving cancer care in our own environment.

Master's Theses

The theses are the most feared part of this study program because they demand a certain level of self-organization, networking, and, of course, scientific work. If students do not have direct patient contact, I strongly encourage them to perform a systematic review on a clinically meaningful question. The systematic reviews should be covering topics that are of interest to the students, but sometimes, a supervisor may have ideas for a thesis project, too. The other appeal of the systematic reviews is that they can be performed everywhere in the world, no matter the own resources. This introduces an aspect of fairness and equality. As long as all parties agree, this will move into the correct direction.

The educational achievement of the completed thesis equals 15 ECTS or a workload of about 450 h. This means that the work must be planned well in advance. Successful completion of the thesis means also that the student is willing to engage in a scientific discussion with the supervisor and vice versa. Even though this is usually the case, there are exceptions on both sides, which may result in a lower satisfaction on either side. Again, communication is key to success as is applied to project management and sometimes escalation.

In many countries, producing an own scientific work is not mandatory to graduate from medical school or its equivalent. Considering the ever-increasing new evidence and the need for critical appraisal of the published literature and ideally distilling the essence of a paper become essential tools for a physician to guide a patient through their cancer journey without harming them. Therefore, I think that unless somebody has access to a larger dataset, the skillset acquired while performing a systematic review is suited best to provide the best possible care for the patients, also in LMICs.

COVID-19-Related Adjustments

As a blended learning study program, we have only little in-person interaction with our students. The highlight of the year is usually the summer seminar at the Reisensburg castle near Günzburg, a secluded venue that enables scientific exchange and networking.

Due to the pandemic, this highlight of the year, together with the originally planned ten-year anniversary alumni meeting, had to be conducted virtually. Also, the ESO-ESMO master class 2020 had to be canceled. All seminars were organized to be conducted virtually, but we realized that sitting in front of a computer can be extremely draining when forced for longer periods. Our communication and negotiation trainers adjusted; our lecturers on pathology, health economic assessments, and evidence-based pathology adjusted; and the virtual format became the new "normal." Also, the workshop on molecular diagnostics was conducted online, and we had the impression that the focus was more toward the explanations than the surroundings making learning enjoyable, too.

In our curriculum, we strive to make learning more palatable by offering more interactions between the seminars. Our psycho-oncologists have devised an entire new training set for patient-centered communication, and this was conducted online—in line with the new "normal" many of our students face during this pandemic.

Benefits for the University

I have asked above whether there is a benefit for the university in running this study program. My answer to this question will always be a resolute "yes."

In offering this study program to participants from all over the world, the university opens its doors to highly educated and ambitious professionals pursuing the goal of improving cancer care in their personal environment. The university shares the expertise of its lecturers but gains also the reputation when these professionals succeed in their settings. Also, the internationalization, one of the developmental aims of the university, is gradually accomplished. You might ask how this may be the case with this small number of students. The point is that all people involved in the processes linked to this study program hone their skillset for internationality and welcoming diversity and serve as little nuclei of excellence wherever they are.

The study program by itself is worldwide unique. Other study programs exist in the field on basic research into oncology or more clinically oriented, but they are not the same, with a zooming-out perspective of oncology worldwide.

Together with our collaboration partner ESO, we have managed a knowledge transfer by establishing other postgraduate continuing education programs, the Certificate of Competence in Lymphoma and the Certificate of Competence in Breast Cancer.

Based on interactions in this study program, currently two grant applications were deposited. One focuses on improving health care in sub-Saharan Africa by means of vaccination; the other one focuses on improving teaching of evidence-based pathology. The latter would once more prove the expertise of Ulm University in running a postgraduate education for learners interested in improving oncology.

Quality Management and Further Plans

Our quality management is extensive, and many other programs might get along with less. However, we have more than 150 lecturers from all over the world, and we think that they can adapt their lectures to the needs of our students only when they know what is needed by the learners. We therefore encourage our students to give us feedback on every lecture they follow. This means that we collect their feedback and report it back to the lecturers and our superiors.

Internally, we attribute medals (gold, silver, bronze) according to the rating within each module. In our feedback letter to each of the lecturers, we communicate the assessment by the students as well as our rating with differing degrees of emergency for renewal, also depending on the previous update. In my function as scientific director, I also follow recent developments and major communications from international meetings and major printed publications. I assess the feedback also with regard to the didactics employed by the lecturer, and I make detailed suggestions for didactic improvement. The major work therefore is updating the lectures according to newly generated knowledge in the basic sciences, new clinical evidence, new legislation, new behavioral aspects, and didactical refinements. This keeps all of us busy.

Our study program was first fully accredited according to the Bologna criteria in 2012, and it was reaccredited in 2018. This accreditation means that the educational achievement, the 60 ECTS, is fully transferable everywhere in Europe and all other countries that recognize the ECTS.

Taking the ten-year anniversary of the study program as a starting point, the inward and outward communication was majorly overhauled. Instead of a generic person, the face of the study program is now a real student carrying her experience with the study program as a message. Content-wise, the learning platform was updated and received a new "look-and-feel" that makes working with the platform easier, everything now optimized for mobile devices like tablet computers. The latter had only been introduced to the market at the time of the start of the study program and are now widely available and in use.

Starting in autumn 2021, interested parties may attend single module to educate themselves further. Among German, Austrian, and Swiss physicians, there was particular interest in the contents of the modules "Interdisciplinary Oncology" and "Advanced Therapies and Integrated Concepts" while claiming that busy schedules prevented many oncologists from engaging in the study program. The Medical Faculty and the Senate of Ulm University have therefore decided to open these modules so as to allow busy physicians to study particular aspects related to their everyday work. This shall serve also the purpose to further educate the workforce without forcing them to pursue the entire curriculum for better serving their patients while preventing burnout.

Acknowledgments The Advanced Oncology study program of Ulm University was funded by a grant of the Ministry of Science and Education of the Federal State of Baden-Württemberg. It would be impossible to run this program without the dedication of its over 150 lecturers as well as the previous and current core teams. ESO has accommodated our students for the ESO/ESMO master classes in clinical oncology, and we are grateful for this generosity.

Over the years, students were supported with scholarships from ESO, the Ruth and Adolf Merckle endowment fund of Ulm University, the Wieland Bildungswerk, and the Robert Bosch Foundation, an unconditional educational grant by Pfizer and the German Academic Exchange Service (DAAD).

I am grateful to everyone involved in running this program smoothly, to the core Advanced Oncology team, to all of our students, and most of all to my genetic and chosen families for their unwavering support.

References

Dittrich C, Kosty M, Jezdic S, Pyle D, Berardi R, Bergh J et al (2016) ESMO/ASCO recommendations for a global curriculum in medical oncology edition. ESMO Open 2016(1):97. https://doi.org/10.1136/esmoopen-2016

ESMO (2021) Global curriculum website. https://www.esmo.org/career-development/global-curriculum-in-medical-oncology. Accessed 24 Feb 2021

George TJ, Manochakian R, Wood M, Polansky M, Baer A, Grupe A, et al. (2021) Quantitative analysis of oncology professional learning preferences. JCO Oncol Pract 16(2):e155-e165 https://doi.org/10.1200/JOP.18.00731

Hansen HH, Bajorin DF, Muss HB, Purkalne G, Schrijvers D, Stahel R (2004) Recommendations for a global core curriculum in medical oncology. J Clin Oncol 22:4616–4625. https://doi.org/10.1200/JCO.2004.08.134

Hoelzer D, Gale RP (2016) Theodor M Fliedner (1 October 1929-9 November 2015), transplant pioneer. Bone Marrow Transplant 51:471–472. https://doi.org/10.1038/bmt.2016.1

Weber-Tuckermann A (2016) Obituary for Theodor M. Fliedner. Uni Ulm Intern. https://www.uni-ulm.de/universitaet/hochschulkommunikation/presse-und-oeffentlichkeitsarbeit/aktuelles-thema/trauer-um-altrektor-professor-theodor-fliedner/. Accessed 11 March 2021

World Health Organization (1998) Advisory Committee on Health Research. A research policy agenda for science and technology to support global health development/Advisory Committee on Health Research. https://apps.who.int/iris/handle/10665/65483. Accessed 11 Mar 2021

Yuan L, Powell S (2013) MOOCs and open education: implications for higher education. https://doi.org/10.13140/2.1.5072.8320

Yuan L, Powell S (2015) Partnership model for entrepreneurial innovation in open online learning. E-learning Papers, 41. ISSN 1887-1542. http://e-space.mmu.ac.uk/619528/. Accessed 31 May 2021

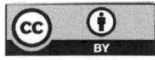

Establishing a Continuing Educational Program Based on the ESMO/ASCO Recommendations for a Global Curriculum in Egypt and Other Educational Initiatives

Zeinab Elsayed, Mohamed Reda Kelany, and Ahmed Magdy Rabea

Revising the Current Curriculum in Clinical Oncology

In Egypt, oncology training programs are either clinical oncology, radiation oncology, or medical oncology (https://www.rcr.ac.uk/clinical-oncology/revalidation. Accessed 2 Feb 2021). Within these programs, candidates are awarded a Master of Science (MSc) degree after three years of training and a Medical Doctorate (MD) after another three training years. For both degrees, the candidate must pass written, clinical, and oral exams together with preparation of an academic medical thesis. The Ministry of Health (MOH) is offering a separate fellowship for radiation oncology and another one for medical oncology in a five-year training. The Children's Cancer Hospital Egypt (57357) has already established a one-year fellowship program in pediatric radia-

tion oncology in collaboration with the Dana-Farber Cancer Institute and Massachusetts General Hospital, Boston, Massachusetts (Bishr and Zaghloul 2018). We have a national standards system for all postgraduate studies (Academic Reference Standards), but we do not have a national board for oncology training.

At the Ain Shams (AS) Clinical Oncology Programs, we have the European Society of Medical Oncology (ESMO), the American Society of Clinical Oncology (ASCO), and the European Society for Therapeutic Radiology and Oncology (ESTRO) recommendations as benchmarks.

This system is different from the UK system in which clinical oncology trainees must complete two years of core medical training and five years of clinical oncology training (https://www.rcr.ac.uk/clinical-oncology/revalidation. Accessed 2 Feb 2021). Our system is also different from that in the USA in which radiation oncology training is a five-year process, while path and training of adult hematology/medical oncology fellows can vary significantly. To enter a fellowship program, candidates must have completed residency training in internal medicine either as categorical or in a combined residency training, such as medicine pediatrics (Knoll 2015).

Z. Elsayed (✉) · M. R. Kelany
Clinical Oncology Department, Ain Shams University Hospitals, Abbassia, Cairo, Egypt
e-mail: z_elsayed@med.asu.edu.eg

A. M. Rabea
Medical Oncology Department, Shefa El Orman Hospital, Luxor, Egypt

Medical Oncology Department, National Cancer Institute, Cairo University, Cairo, Egypt

U. Schmidt-Strassburger (ed.), *Improving Oncology Worldwide*, Sustainable Development Goals Series, https://doi.org/10.1007/978-3-030-96053-7_3

Challenges

As an LMIC, Egypt has several barriers to providing high-quality professional education (Frenk et al. 2010). In the next section, we are going to highlight the most prominent challenges that we face at AS clinical oncology department as an example of oncology departments in university hospitals in Egypt.

Clinical Oncology Curriculum

Clinical oncologists are uncommon in developed countries (apart from the UK) but are the main providers of the service in many LMICs (Popescu et al. 2013). In the past two decades, knowledge has increased rapidly in both radiation oncology and medical oncology specialties, and this makes achieving the necessary competencies in both fields simultaneously very challenging (Sarin 2015). Another problem is that clinical oncologists find it easier to practice the use of systemic therapy than in radiation oncology thereby decreasing in the number of highly qualified radiation oncologists.

Duration of Clinical Oncology Program

Compared to the UK and US programs, the duration of our program is shorter which leads to deficits in training in important parts like research, leadership, communication, and managerial skills. This is also reflected on shortening of other parts in the curriculum as molecular biology and palliative care and spending most of the training time on treating patients with solid tumors.

Limited Resources

Establishing competency-based radiation oncology programs in LMICs is hindered by a lack of resources such as state-of-the-art radiotherapy machines, highly qualified radiation oncologists, and supporting staff (Khader et al. 2020). At the AS clinical oncology department, we have two linear accelerators (one of them is volumetric modulated arc therapy), a CT simulator and an eclipse planning system (with five stations). There is no brachytherapy machine as of this date (due to be launched in April 2021). This infrastructure makes training approximately 15 candidates at different educational stages at a time challenging. We have around 20–25 monthly cases treated by intensity-modulated radiotherapy (IMRT), while the majority of patients receive three-dimensional conformal radiotherapy.

Systemic therapy at the department is sponsored by the Egyptian Ministry of Health (MOH). As other university hospitals and as a country with limited resources, many drugs—especially targeted and immunotherapy—are not covered. These drugs are available in the private sector and some of the health insurance-run hospitals. The safe use of these drugs and management of their side effects constitute an essential part of the clinical oncology training. The present situation makes parts of the curriculum only theoretical with regard to clinical application and thereby incomplete.

Supervision of Trainees

Lack of a structured workplace-based assessment (WPBA) is a very serious problem of the program. This is due to a combination of factors such as limited time of supervisors, lack of faculty training, and resistance of trainees.

Busy Hospital Environment

Egypt has the third largest population in Africa (> 100,000,000) and that makes public and university hospitals very crowded and busy with high volumes of patients and a limited number of supporting staff. At the AS clinical oncology department, we have around 200–250 visiting patients every day. As the system is very hierarchical, trainees are burdened with most of the work, which makes training and feedback very difficult.

Burnout

Burnout and the inability to have a healthy work-life balance are the most serious challenges in our working environment. According to a recently published survey study at the AS clinical oncology department, 72% of participants (52 clinical oncologists) had burnout on the emotional exhaustion (EE) scale, 49% on the depersonalization (DP) scale, and 38% on the personal accomplishment (PA) scale (Ghali et al. 2019).

Lack of Research Opportunities

Limited budgets for research together with time constraints and lack of a reasonable number of international clinical trials at the department make trainees lack the opportunity to publish in high-impact specialized medical journals.

Assessment System

Our current assessment system is a pass-fail system (at 60%) and summative. It enforces focusing on knowledge rather than skills and lacks the very important part of "feedback." Candidates have one final exam at the end of their training. Lack of frequent formative assessment is a serious problem with the current program as it makes the continuous professional development at this early career stage less transparent and less encouraging.

Chances

Residents

While the described challenges are eminent, the biggest resources are the physicians themselves, their ties to the country, and their eagerness to perform. This is particularly true for graduates from Ain Shams (AS) University, who are traditionally very competitive and have high aspirations with regard to their own performance, but also with regard to supporting infrastructure. The decision to care for oncology patients oftentimes comes from a biographical background and therefore is a very strong motivator to perform and to perform best. We already have many physicians—trained within this system—who transferred to the USA and Europe and are doing very well. We have also many other successful graduates who chose to continue in their country and contribute to the advance of AS University in the international ranking with their publications.

Educators

Ambitious students and residents may sometimes challenge established pathways. Even though this may be perceived as a threat by some individuals, the possibilities are that faculty is adopting new knowledge and new ways of conduct thereby strengthening their own positions by allowing innovation but also empowering residents and younger faculty. The constant challenge to update one's own knowledge and skillset keeps a young spirit and an ambiance of mutual respect.

The Pathway to Reform

Needs Assessment

Many focus group discussions of the different stakeholder groups together with program evaluation tools revealed the shortcomings of the current program as mentioned above. We conducted these discussions between residents and educators encouraging an exchange.

A Separate Radiation Oncology and Medical Oncology Curriculum

As a result, the separation between the two specialties seems inevitable. The ESMO/ASCO Global Curriculum for Training in Medical Oncology is one of the benchmarks of AS clinical oncology program, but it cannot be applied in the current situation. Separating the two specialties will allow the proper implementation of this curriculum. The ESTRO Core Curriculum for Radiation Oncology/Radiotherapy will be one of the main benchmarks for our Radiation Oncology curriculum. Community and cultural issues must be taken into consideration. All stakeholders will be invited to participate. It is of utmost importance to keep the ties that were historically established in order to provide residents with the best training according to their interest as well as the patients with the best comprehensive care possible.

National and International Collaboration

Collaborating with both national and international bodies is very important. Sharing of resources and expertise will enhance high-quality radiation oncology education. The Ulm Master Degree in Advanced Oncology is a very good example of how international collaboration can help LMICs in faculty development. Implementing the ESMO/ASCO curriculum with the help of ASCO outreach for international programs will be the next step in adapting a blueprint for postgraduate education of medical professionals in Egypt.

Faculty Development

In a period of change, open communication is key to a successful implementation of the envisaged changes. Therefore, training staff on WPBA and mentorship is crucial. One option to achieve this objective would be to enroll in international mentorship programs available free of charge, for example, of the European School of Oncology or to send residents and faculty to respective mentorship programs of the ESMO or the ASCO.

Change the Current Assessment System

In order to change the current system of assessment and to make its outcome more transparent to all parties involved, a portfolio and WPBA must be implemented. Continuous formative assessment and remediation strategies must be endorsed, and the ACGME Milestones for Hematology and Oncology provide excellent guidance for this purpose (Collichio and Muchmore 2018). It is essential to assess resident's performance regularly and to give feedback, also 360° feedback, without fearing repercussions from any party involved in the process.

In summary, all these processes are aimed at improving the current procedures and pathways by professionalizing continuing education of our oncology and radiotherapy residents and thereby providing a mutually beneficial atmosphere of respect, trust, and quality.

Establishing a Sarcoma Program in Egypt

Sarcomas are very rare tumors and very heterogeneous, and their treatment is particularly challenging since it demands a high level of cooperation between different medical and non-medical subspecialties. Even the official site on cancer statistics, the Global Cancer Observatory (www.gco.iarc.fr), does not issue fact sheets for sarcomas other than Kaposi's sarcoma, a disease associated with HIV infection (Bray et al. 2018).

Egypt had completely lacking incidence rates at the national level until the development of the National Cancer Registry Program of Egypt (NCRPE) in 2008. The NCRPE stratified Egypt into three geographical strata: lower, middle, and upper. A recent publication from NCRPE based upon the incidence rates of cancer in Egypt in 2008–2011 revealed that "the crude incidence rates for all cancer sites excluding non-melanoma skin cancer were 113.1/100,000. Soft tissue sarcoma crude incidence is 2.2/100,000 for the male population and 1.9/100,000 for the female population (Ibrahim et al. 2014).

Finishing the Advanced Oncology study program at Ulm University strengthened the desire to establish an Egyptian soft tissue sarcoma

Table 1 Strengths, weaknesses, opportunities, and threats of the proposed Egyptian sarcoma network

Strength	Weakness	Opportunity	Threat
• Manpower • Patient numbers	• The quality of data collection and storage • Lacking tissue banking • Less collaboration • Wide range of health-care facilities	• We have well-established research units and ethical review committees	• Logistics pathways take long times • Lack of funding • Cultural issues • Fear of change issues

network. On one hand, we have the patients with their challenging diseases; on the other hand, the treating physicians might feel the need to double-check their treatment decisions with equally educated and experienced other professionals. Even though everybody is working hard and is an avid reader of the scientific literature, the differences in health-care provision and reimbursement might pose an additional challenge for the physicians, but most definitely also for the patients and their families.

Despite increasing evidence supporting a referral to specialized sarcoma units, most of our patients are not managed according to guidelines, particularly those in the early stage of their disease requiring surgery.

Here in Egypt, we have a lot of great minds and hard workers, but they work separately in different national-based oncology centers or privately based within a very wide range of different health-care facilities like separate islands lacking from bridges or power collaboration between them, which affects the outcome (less so-called effective outcome) and also significantly affects the research work and the international clinical trial involvement. So, despite these great single workers, we still remain in a dark zone internationally.

Focusing in one cancer subtype (sarcoma) is my dream to create a national sarcoma network aiming for a better clinical registry also for better pathological diagnosis using molecular pathology as well as improving the surgical and overall outcomes.

The goal is to reach the true multidisciplinary approach in managing individual malignancies and establishing formal training based on the ASCO/ESMO Task Force on the Global Core Curriculum in Medical Oncology with collabora-

tion with various major specialties such as surgery, radiotherapy, and pathology (Hansen et al. 2008). This a step further, creating an adaptive national guideline in oncological management of soft tissue sarcoma and creating a well-developed nest with tissue banking to participate in international clinical trials globally (Table 1).

Only joint action and education on the different topics can overcome the current weaknesses and threats. The benefit for patients and society must be clearly communicated and involve patient advocate groups as well as different stakeholders for the scientific societies representing the disciplines involved in the management of patients with sarcomas.

Challenges that Need to be Met

I am a medical oncologist from Egypt and one of the first graduates of the Advanced Oncology study program. The curriculum seemed and still seems to help in my career as a faculty member in the National Cancer Institute of Egypt, where I am a lecturer and consultant of Medical Oncology and Hematology. The module particularly interesting to me was the one that covered molecular biology during the first semester. Also getting to know physicians from all over the world, staying connected to them to this day, the experience of diversity in the methodology of thinking and collaboration, meeting at international conferences, and keeping a strong relation, particularly with part of the faculty program, changed my professional perspective and finally its trajectory.

I have been using the knowledge and skillset I gained during the master's program in teaching the young residents and fellows. Also, the knowledge I gained helped me a lot in understanding the new treatment modalities and the translational medicine behind it. Currently, I serve as the head of the medical oncology department in a nongovernmental organization hospital called Shefa El Orman Hospital in Luxor, South of Egypt, where we are treating patients for free and accepting fellows and residents whom I am responsible for with regard to their training.

What has been established so far? Weekly educational lectures and daily clinical rounds for residents and fellows bring bench to bedside teaching to these trainees. In addition, twice weekly clinical pharmacists' educational meetings and monthly nursing staff educational meetings ensure proper education of nonmedical professionals involved in the care of oncology patients. Some of our trainees and residents are now residents in the UK, KSA, and UAE, perfecting their training in these countries.

Egypt is a developing country, and there are challenges that need to be addressed and will help in the improvement of the academic level of the hospital and the educational programs currently available. Collaboration with an international body in assisting and guiding the improvement of our current training program and obtaining the accreditation required for this program to be internationally known and applied would help. Also, other developing countries in the region might feel encouraged and empowered by sending their physicians, nurses, and pharmacists for clinical and academic training. This will definitely reduce the cost of traveling and accommodation and widen the locoregional network. Another option would be to collaborate with other internationally oriented academic programs to supply the clinical part of the program which will strengthen the academic program in other faculties and would allow more collaboration between this and other international centers through supplying their academic parts to students and fellows. Also, this can open a collaboration channel for physician exchange programs again helping transfer the Western experience and applying it in other developing countries, which will improve the medical and academic services supplied by other centers.

Considering the busy clinics and difficulties to maintain the clinical and academic parts, bringing more fellows and trainees would help in improving the medical services provided. The fellows from abroad will experience the clinical training required through hands-on experience, real-life data, and not only academic education. Afterward, they can transfer the knowledge that they have acquired to their own countries and faculties thereby starting their own educational programs. Hoping for a domino effect, this might lead to a huge collaborative educational body in the region and will allow for clinical trials and research to be applied.

The educational program provided at my current Shefa El Orman Hospital is similar in many points to the curriculum recommended by ESMO/ASCO. Using the ESMO/ASCO logbook, benchmarking (Hansen et al. 2008) was performed, and efforts to implement the Egyptian curriculum for future use and to accredit this program are underway. So far, the Egyptian board of medical oncology approved hosting of residents, and enlistment by the UICC (Union for International Cancer Control) has been completed. The whole medical team, the board of directors, and the pharmaceutical companies have supported educational events with very much enthusiasm.

If this model succeeds and receives the deserved recognition, our project's blueprint can be used as a model for other faculties and centers allowing improvement of the oncology services available to our patients.

Acknowledgments ZE and AMR were supported by the European School of Oncology (ESO) for participating in the Advanced Oncology study program of Ulm University. MRK received a scholarship grant from the Ruth and Adolf Merckle endowment fund at the Ulm University foundation.

References

Bishr MK, Zaghloul MS (2018) Radiation therapy availability in Africa and Latin America: two models of low and middle income countries. Int J Radiat Oncol Biol Phys 102(3):490–498. https://doi.org/10.1016/j.ijrobp.2018.06.046. Epub 2018 Jul 10

Bray F, Ferlay J, Soerjomataram I, Siegel RL, Torre LA, Jemal A (2018) Global cancer statistics 2018: GLOBOCAN estimates of incidence and mortality worldwide for 36 cancers in 185 countries. CA Cancer J Clin 68(6):394–424

Collichio F, Muchmore EA (2018) The American Society of Hematology and ASCO curricular milestones for assessment of fellows in hematology/oncology: development, reflection, and next steps. Am Soc Clin Oncol Educ Book 38:887–893

Frenk J, Chen L, Bhutta ZA et al (2010) Health professionals for a new century: trans-forming education to strengthen health systems in an interdependent world. Lancet 376(9756):1923–1958. https://doi.org/10.1016/S0140-6736(10)61854-5. PMID: 21112623

Ghali R, Boulos D, Alorabi M (2019) Cross-sectional study of burnout among a Group of Egyptian Oncologists at Ain Shams University. Res Oncol 15(1):26–30. https://doi.org/10.21608/resoncol.2018.3478.1056

Hansen HH, Bajorin DF, Muss HB, Purkalne G, Schrijvers D, Stahel R. ESMO-ASCO global Core curriculum for training in medical oncology log book. 2008.. https://www.esmo.org/content/download/8176/168808/file/The-ESMO-ASCO-Global-Core-Curriculum-for-Training-in-Medical-Oncology-Log-Book.pdf. Accessed 28 May 2021

Ibrahim AS, Khaled HM, Mikhail NN, Baraka H, Kamel H (2014) Cancer incidence in Egypt: results of the national population-based cancer registry program. J Cancer Epidemiol 2014:437971

Khader J, Al-Mousa A, Al Khatib S et al (2020) Successful development of a competency-based residency training program in radiation oncology: our 15-year experience from within a developing country. J Canc Educ 35:1011–1016. https://doi.org/10.1007/s13187-019-01557-8

Knoll, M., 2015. Contemporary clinical oncology training in the United States: is radiation or medical oncology right for you? [Blog] ASCO Connection. https://connection.asco.org/blogs/contemporary-clinical-oncology-training-united-states-radiation-or-medical-oncology-right-you. Accessed 3 Feb 2021

Popescu RA, Schäfer R, Califano R et al (2013) The current and future role of the medical oncologist in the professional care for cancer patients: a position paper by the European Society for Medical Oncology (ESMO). Ann Oncol 25(1):9–15. https://doi.org/10.1093/annonc/mdt522. PMID: 24335854

Sarin R (2015) Global trends in specialist training, certification, and regulation of oncology practice and its implications for the developing world. J Cancer Res Ther 11(4):675–678. https://doi.org/10.4103/0973-1482.176090

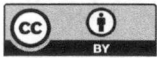

Continuing Education for the Young Oncology Workforce in Portugal

Judy Vicente de Paulo

Introduction

Oncology is a field of medicine dedicated to prevention, diagnosis, staging, treatment, and follow-up of patients with malignant neoplasms and their complications, as well as to palliative and supportive care. The medical oncologist, in addition to the crucial role they play in monitoring of the cancer patient, should be able to understand the natural history, biology, and genetics of cancer and the principles of its treatment; prevent and diagnose stage cancer and malignant diseases; decide and propose the appropriate therapies; execute the various modalities of medical treatment of neoplasms, as well as assessing and controlling their side effects, throughout the evolution of the different tumors, including the terminal stage of the disease, in ambulatory and/or inpatient, as well as in an individual, family, social, and professional context through close communication with their patients and family members; and outline, conduct, and interpret clinical and/or laboratory research studies (Dittrich et al. 2016;

Portuguese Oncology Society 2021; Nucleus of Young Oncologists 2021).

The Situation in Portugal

In fact, medical oncology in Portugal was for years a sub-specialization of internal medicine residency, but nowadays, it is a five-year specialization comprising internships of oncology, internal medicine, intensive medicine, hematology, and radio-oncology along with a research project development.

As worldwide, residency is demanding, clinically, scientifically, and personally, and most of the residents embrace it with a profound dedication and commitment, as medical oncology covers more than the disease itself and its treatment. This specialty sees the patient as a whole, integrating psychological, social, and spiritual aspects, namely, in the constant confrontation with the threat at the end of life. As such, medical oncology is a challenge for all healthcare professionals, the complexity of its pathophysiology, the constant increase in scientific knowledge, and the countless hopeful therapeutic strategies that are discovered every day.

It does not make sense to talk about medical oncology without talking about multidisciplinary teamwork, dedicated and prepared to embrace the patients and the disease in all their aspects. This feature is an added value to any physician,

J. V. de Paulo (✉)
Portuguese Insitute of Oncology of Coimbra, Coimbra, Portugal

U. Schmidt-Strassburger (ed.), *Improving Oncology Worldwide*, Sustainable Development Goals Series, https://doi.org/10.1007/978-3-030-96053-7_4

having the privilege of sharing and discussing cases and learning from their peers every day. On the other hand, research in oncology underlies our daily practice in either basic, translational, and clinical research, being also an important mark of medical oncology residency.

All in all, gathering all the complexity of this branch of medicine, along with the challenging path of the residency, little time remains for theoretical education.

Therefore, the importance of gathering experiences and knowledge within residents and young oncologists led to an informal meeting between oncology youngsters aiming to support the education and networking of residents and young oncologists in Portugal.

The Nucleus of Interns and Young Specialists (NIJE)

In 2014, a group of young residents organized a national medical oncology residents' meeting and that generated the need for creating a Young Oncologists Committee.

The Nucleus of Interns and Young Specialists (NIJE) of the Portuguese Society of Oncology (SPO) was born in 2015 firstly through an installer group which was followed in 2016 by the first official NIJE of SPO in which I had the pleasure to participate (Portuguese Oncology Society 2021; Nucleus of Young Oncologists 2021). Gradually, and with the unconditional support of the SPO's presidency, this committee created events, courses, and new initiatives, always with the objective of improving training in oncology in Portugal and bringing together the younger generations of this field.

NIJE is composed of interns and young specialists (under the age of 40 years old) from different regions of the country, aiming to represent all the young oncologists nationwide and collecting their opinions, suggestions, or concerns facilitating the active participation of all in NIJE.

One of NIJE's main objectives was to actively monitor the training process of residents in Portugal as well as to create continuous training actions promoting postgraduate courses and other complementary training actions in oncology.

From 2016 throughout 2018, nowadays still growing, training courses were held on a monthly basis as part of the "8 months 8 courses" project. These courses were designed to cover the main areas lacking formation during residency, a welcome course, a master class covering all cancer types, training skills in communication, statistics, oncological emergencies, formation in cancer research, support and palliative care, and more recently medical writing.

In more detail, a brief description of each NIJE initiative is discussed.

In-Person Meetings and Trainings

The **Course of Introduction to the Specialty of Medical Oncology**, started in 2015, intends to welcome the interns of the first year of Medical Oncology residency program and addresses topics such as the presentation of the SPO and NIJE, description of the structure of the Medical Oncology Internship, share of bibliography in oncology, and the main oncology-related organizations in a day intended to promote networking. Additionally, we offered three short tutorial talks: "How to manage a database" Workshop, "How to compose a successful abstract," and "How to survive a residency," the latter covering important topics such as burnout in oncology healthcare professionals, mainly in residents.

The **SPO Oncology Course** is an initiative that aims a qualified education of interns in medical oncology, with a special focus on interns in more advanced phases of training. With this course, interns receive didactic training on basic mechanisms of cell growth, pharmacology, and theoretical bases of chemotherapy and indications and management of toxicities of systemic treatments in the various areas of oncology. They also have the possibility to discuss clinical cases interactively, with the support of voting by televote. In order to consolidate all knowledge, the interns have a final evaluation test. The video support of the lectures (sent after the course in digital format) allows interns and young specialists to revisit the lectures and maintain the "continuous learning" model. During the week, a group of 35 trainees have social moments during the week where networking and sharing experiences and knowledge are privileged.

The **Oncology Communication Course** is a training activity with several stations/role-plays that addresses the communication process involved in oncology practice. Topics cover communicating bad news, framing prognostic information to both patient and families, managing emotions, and communication in transition of care or end of life. This significant competence is often underestimated in our academic formation, and skills must be given to strengthen the medical-patient relationship and minimize burnout risks.

The **Statistics Course** was organized by NIJE/SPO in collaboration with the Association for University Extension of the Faculty of Economics of the University of Coimbra (APEU/FEUC). This course intends to assist health professionals to identify, apply, analyze, and interpret fundamental statistical procedures, which include descriptive statistics, inferential statistics, and multivariate analyses using the SPSS® statistical software. With a strong practical component, databases of own research work were discussed and suggested by NIJE members, complementing the theoretical part with a hands-on component. The aim of this course is to increase statistical knowledge in young residents in order to improve not only the interpretation of scientific publications but also with regard to a scientific project's quality.

In a different format, **the Oncology Emergencies/Critical Patient Course** aimed to enhance the trainees' skills in addressing oncology emergencies as well as promoting the discussion of practical cases and discussing the referral of cancer patients to intensive and intermediate care units. On the first day of the course, we had the support of a digital interactive simulator (Body Interact) simulating clinical cases of emergencies in clinical cases of pulmonary thromboembolism and pericardial tamponade thanks to a partnership with a local company of technology for clinical education. On the second day, some of the authors of the "Recommendations for intensive medical treatment in cancer patients," endorsed by a SPO's working group, were brought together with an important reflection on the decisions to be made in each situation, in a sharing environment of experiences.

The application to **the Cancer Research Course** was made through a research project and the candidates' curriculum vitae. During the course, each participant was assigned to a mentor, and the research projects were discussed and refined for resubmission for a grant application. Thus, in addition to providing a theoretical component about different types of cancer research (basic, translational, and clinical), this course helps the participant, in a more practical component, with the construction of correctly designed research projects, increasing the quality of research from the early stages of the training of young oncologists. These trainee's/trainer's meetings were scheduled over the three-day course. At the end of the course, four scholarships were awarded to the four most innovative projects in oncology. Through these grants, we want to encourage and support scientific research, linking national and international networks of researchers and gathering young interns and basic research institutions.

The **Supportive and Palliative Care Course** is a partnership with the Portuguese Association of Palliative Care and counts with the participation of a representative of ESMO Designated Centres Working Group (DCWG). This course offers an overall perspective of important topics on supportive and palliative care, an area of extreme importance in all oncology specialties lacks integrated training during the internship. Training in supportive therapies is crucial in medical training in oncology, namely, the approach to pain, as well as the early integration of palliative care. Thus, union and representation of the various associations are essential to encompass the complexity and multidisciplinary teamwork that this topic requires in two days of full sharing of knowledge.

Online Initiatives

Moreover, several online initiatives took place in order to support our motto of formation "anytime anywhere." The webinars of clinical cases in oncology were streaming webinars with clinical discussion between a NIJE member and an invited oncologist and encouraged the debate of daily practice clinical cases. The NIJE member and the specialist discuss the various steps in the diagnosis staging and treatment of the various oncological pathologies. The video teaser was available online, but only SPO members can watch the webinar in its entirety.

Also, in innovation of the SPO, a website was introduced by the Young Oncologists Corner. The narrowing of NIJE/Young Oncologists links with ESMO and the creation of the platform "Portuguese oncologists around the world" were other important steps. The platform on the SPO website of the "Portuguese oncologists around the world" allows the dissemination of information for health professionals or Portuguese researchers in oncology who are working outside our country, with the objective of sharing experiences between peers and colleagues who wish to undertake fellowships outside Portugal. A form was sent to the subscribers to agree to make available, allowing, in accordance with confidentiality rules, to provide the name, institution, and areas of oncology in which they are working abroad. Those interested in contact with the listed elements contact the SPO, which will provide (after permission from the international party) the email address, thereby promoting network and involving the stakeholders abroad in a national project.

COVID-Related Adjustments

The online extension of the courses, having been planned before, was accelerated with the current global status due to the pandemic of COVID-19. After the months of March 2020, an online training platform (Moodle platform) was designed, from young people for young people, to continue the training for the youngest in oncology, since all the clinical activities and internships must continue despite the huge impact of COVID-19 pandemic in our professional and personal lives. Underlining that the objective of these courses is always networking, reinforcing physical presence (as soon as possible again), the first e-learning Course on Support and Palliative Care and the first e-learning Investigation Course were launched. We also counted on the partnership with PALOPS (Portuguese-speaking African countries) interns and young specialists with free enrollment in the courses. Privileging the "continuous learning model, without losing the networking component," the training blocks were made available to the trainees during a week, with a "live" session via videoconference with some of the speakers answering questions and discussing hot topics on the last day of the course.

In addition, there is an enormous commitment to involve all specialties related to oncology—medical oncology, radio-oncology, and surgical oncology—and to link SPO to ESMO by linking NIJE to ESMO Young Oncologists Committee, representing and uniting young interns and international specialists (ESMO 2021).

Conclusion

In short, NIJE and SPO aim to be a reference in the training of young residents in the various specialties in oncology through "continuous learning," as well as to encourage and support scientific research, contributing to network among young oncologists in Portugal.

Above all, this recent Young Oncologists group aims to unite interns and young specialists in oncology, encouraging teamwork and interrelationship and sharing of clinical, training, and investigative experiences, thus promoting emotional wellness during residency and enlarging the quality of oncology in Portugal.

Acknowledgments NIJE is grateful to the ongoing support by the SPO and unconditional educational grants from the pharmaceutical industry. Without this financial support, the training would not have been possible.

References

Dittrich C, Kosty M, Jezdic S et al (2016) ESMO/ASCO Recommendations for a Global Curriculum in Medical Oncology Edition 2016. Open 1:97

ESMO (2021) Young Oncologists Committee. https://www.esmo.org/about-esmo/organisational-structure/young-oncologists-committee. Accessed 30 Jun 2021.

Nucleus of Young Oncologists (2021) https://www.spon-cologia.pt/pt/jovens-oncologistas/nucleo-de-jovens/. Accessed 30 Jun 2021.

Portuguese Oncology Society (2021) https://www.spon-cologia.pt/pt/. Accessed 30 Jun 2021.

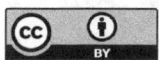

Challenges and Outcomes in Launching the First Board-Certified Program in Radiation Oncology in Iraq

Layth Mula-Hussain

Background

Board-certified residency programs are essential for safe and competent practice in any medical specialty, including radiation oncology. In some countries, these specialty training programs are not yet established (Mula-Hussain et al. 2021). This chapter describes how, despite the political, economic, and social obstacles, the first board-certified residency program in radiation oncology was successfully launched in Iraq during 2013–2017. The result was the work of many, especially my co-authors of the earlier versions of this report. The effort would not have been possible without the public fund through the Ministry of Health at the Kurdistan Regional Government in Iraq and the support of the Kurdistan Board for Medical Specialties (KBMS), besides additional support from many private and not-for-profit authorities and individuals.

By definition, radiation oncology is the discipline of clinical medicine that uses ionizing radi-

ation, either alone or in combination with other modalities, to treat patients with malignant diseases (mostly) or nonmalignant conditions (occasionally) (International Atomic Energy Agency 2009). The common cancers controlled by radiotherapy are the prostate, lung, rectum, uterus, head, and neck and many other sites. Of those cancer patients who are cured, it is estimated that 49% are cured by surgery, about 40% by radiotherapy alone or combined with other modalities, and 11% by chemotherapy alone or combined (International Atomic Energy Agency 2017).

The first establishment of radiotherapy services in Iraq dates back to the 1920s when the Radiology Institute was established in Baghdad (Al-Ghazi 2016). This institute was the only place in Iraq offering radiation services until the late 1950s when a deep X-ray therapy unit was installed in Mosul in 1959. The Iraqi pioneers in this field got governmental scholarships to complete their specialty programs in the UK. After their return, and similar to the British training program in the 1960s–1970s, the College of Medicine at the University of Baghdad established the first specialty program in Iraq (two-year DMRT) in 1985 (Mula-Hussain 2012). These early initiatives came before many similar developments in the nearby countries to Iraq (Mula-Hussain et al. 2019c). Unfortunately, the progress discontinued due to wars and its consequences that Iraq passed through from the 1990s onward, where many professionals left the coun-

An earlier version of this material was presented originally at the 2019 Annual Scientific Meeting of the Canadian Association of Radiation Oncology, Halifax, NS, CANADA (Mula-Hussain et al. 2019a); and published at the Clinical and Translational Radiation Oncology 19 (2019) 46–51 (Mula-Hussain et al. 2019b).

L. Mula-Hussain (✉)
Radiation Oncology, College of Medicine—Ninevah University, Mosul, Iraq

© The Author(s) 2022
U. Schmidt-Strassburger (ed.), *Improving Oncology Worldwide*, Sustainable Development Goals Series,
https://doi.org/10.1007/978-3-030-96053-7_5

try and development was halted by the embargo and sanctions, which further increased by the occupation in 2003. In 2010, there were only about 30 radiation (or clinical) oncologists and 6 megavoltage machines (MVMs, which are the machines used in radiotherapy) in the whole country. This small number supposed to serve over 32 million Iraqis and around 20 thousand new cancer patients at that time (Mula-Hussain 2012). The resulting ratio of less than one radiation oncologist for every million population is about a tenth of the recommended staffing ratio in other countries (usually 8–12 radiation oncologists per million) (International Atomic Energy Agency 2010).

I describe the challenges and outcomes associated with the establishment of the first board-certified radiation oncology program in Iraq during the period 2013–2017, including the steps that were taken to overcome the challenges. This effort may serve as a mirror for other colleagues trying to establish such educational programs in their countries.

Challenges and Baseline Status

Recognition of the Obstacles

The obstacles in establishing a board-certified radiation oncology program in Iraq were due, but not limited, to lack, or insufficiency, of (1) qualified board-certified trainers in radiation oncology; (2) clinical training centers; (3) modern equipment with required maintenance; (4) quality assurance measures in radiation oncology; (5) academic education, accreditation, and certification; (6) administrative support; (7) financial support; (8) political stability; (9) scientific and professional connectedness; and (10) straightforward bureaucratic processes.

Baseline Status of the Radiotherapy Center

The Zhianawa Cancer Center (ZCC) is a public, tertiary cancer care facility in Sulaimani City (360 km northeast to Baghdad and 200 km east to Erbil, Fig. 1). ZCC is a dedicated center for radiotherapy, established in 2009. Its services are free of charge and open to all Iraqis (Zhianawa Cancer Center 2017). ZCC was initially staffed by two specialists in radiation oncology with eight residents. These junior resident physicians were enrolled in this center after passing the center's requirements during the period from 2009 through 2012. Unfortunately, they stayed without recognition as the center was not yet staffed with qualified trainer(s) in radiation oncology. The residents needed structured academic and practical guidance to become certified specialists and practice independently and safely.

Overcoming the Challenges

Part I: Defining the Structured Training Program

Contract Agreement with an External Qualified Radiation Oncology Trainer

As many professionals left the country from the 1990s onward, it was impossible to establish an advanced (board-level) program in this field without the availability of a single board-certified radiation oncology trainer locally (Mula-Hussain and Al-Ghazi 2020). Radiation oncology is a complex clinical field and requires well-trained personnel. Investment in personnel should precede that in equipment to achieve a satisfactory outcome. Based on this, the first step was to choose a board-certified person from abroad and qualified to lead the effort of establishing such a program locally. To achieve this goal, ZCC in Sulaimani started to contact external trainers during the 2010s. Eventually, the officials from the Regional Ministry of Health signed a four-year contract with an external trainer (the author of this chapter).

The local leaders of ZCC invited this external trainer to visit the center in 2011 to address its suitability for the postgraduate accredited training program. The visitor examined the infrastructure and the available human and equipment resources. He wrote a visit report with recom-

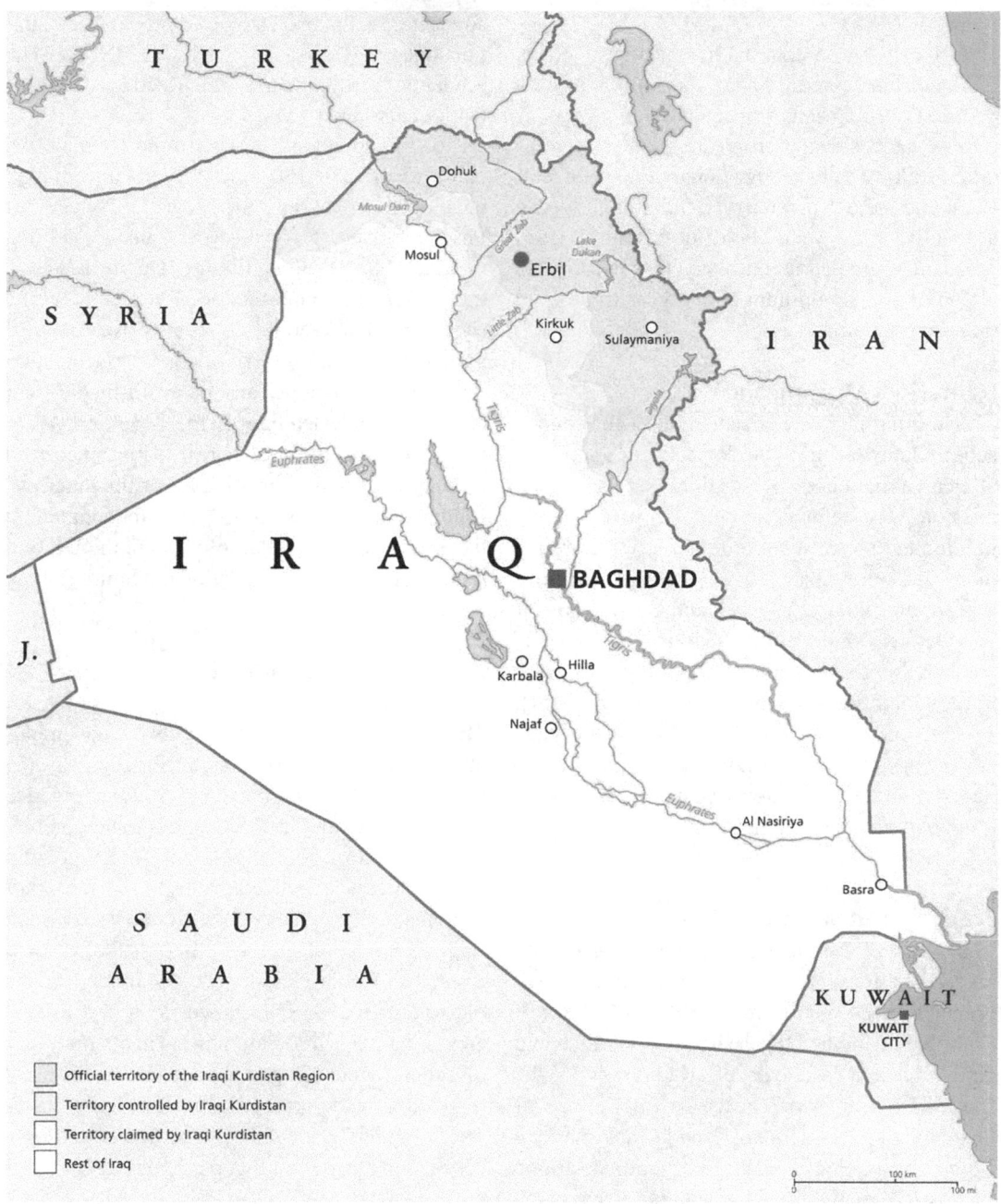

Fig. 1 Sulaimani (Sulaymaniyah) and its relation to the federal capital (Baghdad) and the regional capital (Erbil), northeast of Iraq. Both cities are part of Kurdistan. J.: Jordan. Source: Getty Images

mendations to update the available equipment resources and a roadmap for moving forward. This visit was also coupled with meeting the academic leadership team at the KBMS to meet their organizational requirements in postgraduate medical education and recognition. After about 18 months from the visit report and following the recommendations, the external trainer returned to ZCC to start the in-house training process in the second quarter of 2013.

Accreditations

With the in-house external trainer's availability, ZCC got the accreditation of the KBMS to be a certified training center in radiation oncology for a four-year residency program. Another accreditation followed this recognition by the College of Medicine—the University of Sulaimani for an alternative three-year Master of Science (MSc) program in radiation oncology (for those who already have a minimum of one-year training in radiation oncology).

Definition, Mission, and Vision

The training pathway is settled to let the trainee acquire knowledge in oncologic science and gain clinical experience in radiation oncology. The mission was defined as "serving patients, the public, and the medical profession by certifying that ZCC diplomates have acquired, demonstrated, and maintained the requisite standard of knowledge, skill, understanding, and performance essential to the safe and competent practice of radiation oncology" (Datta et al. 2014). The vision is that by 2020, ZCC will have advanced safety and quality in healthcare by setting definitive professional standards for radiation oncology (Mula-Hussain 2013), which it has achieved.

Training and Study Syllabus

The syllabus was devised using well-structured resources in clinical radiation oncology programs, like the syllabi from the Royal College of Radiologists in the UK, the Royal Australian and New Zealand College of Radiologists, the CanMEDS framework of the Royal College of Physicians and Surgeons of Canada, the American Board of Radiology, and the International Atomic Energy Agency (IAEA) syllabus that was endorsed by the American Society for Therapeutic Radiology and Oncology (ASTRO) and the European Society for Therapeutic Radiology and Oncology (ESTRO). There were 10 modules, with 100 credits over 4 years in the KBMS board program and 75 credits over 3 years in the university MSc program. The residents have to achieve the seven competency requirements (medical experts, communicators, collaborators, leaders,

advocates, scholars, and professionals in radiation oncology, as defined by CanMEDS). The academic credits are summarized in Table 1 (Mula-Hussain 2013).

For the length of the structured training, we opted to make it full-time 4 years in radiation oncology, following the Royal College of Physicians and Surgeons of Canada and the American Board of Radiology. Due to administrative logistics and the need to increase the acceptance but keeping the quality, we designed an alternative pathway of specialty certification through the university and of a full-time 3-year course of study leading to the MSc degree for those who already have 1 year of uncategorized training in radiation oncology. For the latter, we followed the well-established syllabi adopted by the Royal College of Radiologists in the UK and the IAEA syllabus (International Atomic Energy Agency 2009).

Admission and Academic Requirements

The main admission requirements include graduation from a recognized medical school by the ministry of higher education, hold a practice license by the medical association, and completion of a rotatory general residency of a minimum of 12 months. Applicants must pass the entry examination in oncology foundations, be good English users, and successfully pass the personal interview (Mula-Hussain 2013). Each trainee must publish a paper in a peer-reviewed journal and/or complete a research thesis in the final year of training. According to the board and university regulations, every specialist needs to show scientific merit and critical appraisal before getting a certification degree in that particular field.

Clinical Training (Major and Minor Rotations)

Under supervision, residents rotate in four groups, two residents each, sequentially. Each major rotation has a duration of 3 months in radiation oncology and is repeated three to four times during the studies with increasing independence granted to residents as their skills develop. During each rotation, the resident passes through

Table 1 Academic disciplines, didactic and practical hours, and equivalent credits (Mula-Hussain 2013)

	Academic disciplines (modules)	Training hours		Credits[a] (D/P)
		Didactic (D)	Practical (P)	
1.	Cancer biology and radiation biology	45 (first Y)	0	3
2.	Medical physics	45 (first Y)	135 (1st–second Y)	6 (3 + 3)
3.	Medical research and cancer epidemiology	45 (first Y)	0	3
4.	Onco-pharmacology	30 (first Y)	0	2
5.	Radiological anatomy and diagnostic oncology	30 (first Y)	45 (first Y)	3 (2 + 1)
6.	Tumor pathology and laboratory	30 (first Y)	45 (first Y)	3 (2 + 1)
7.	Medical oncology	30 (second Y)	90 (second Y)	4 (2 + 2)
8.	Surgical oncology	15 (second Y)	45 (second Y)	2 (1 + 1)
9.	Clinical radiation oncology	75 (1st–third Y)	2655[b] (1st–fourth Y)	64 (5 + 59)
10.	Academic work	30 (third Y)	360 (third Y)	10 (2 + 8)
		375	**3375**	**100 (25D + 75 P)**

Notes

[a] One credit equals 15 didactic hours (1 h/week for 15 weeks) or 45 practical hours (3 h/week for 15 weeks),

[b] 2655 h distributed as 500, 750, 750, and 655 annual hours during the first, second, third, and fourth year, respectively,

One-hundred credits for the four-year KBMS board program and 75 credits for the three-year university MSc program (similarly 375 didactic hours, correspondingly proportionate practical hours)

new patients' clinics, on-treatment clinics, post-treatment follow-up clinics, simulation techniques, volumes' contouring, and plan evaluation sessions. Minor rotations were arranged, too, each of 2–4 weeks duration, in diagnostic radiology, tumor pathology, medical oncology, surgical oncology, palliative care, and cancer research (Mula-Hussain 2013).

Evaluation, Promotion, and Examination

A regular evaluation, that is, a written examination and oral assessment, was arranged at the end of each clinical rotation and each didactic course. Annual evaluation (written examination and practical assessment) was organized at the end of each training year. Feedback from all the peers and co-workers was considered. However, the infrastructure so far was not permissive to a 360° review. On campus (at ZCC) and a yearly report were sent to the KBMS and the university about promoting the trainee to the following year. Part one examination was conducted at the KBMS and the university after successful completion of the first year. The final examination took place at the KBMS and university upon successful completion of the last year. A significant guideline for assessment is to see if the candidate demonstrates the competency to practice safely and independently. This examination consisted of two written exams (over 2 days) and an oral and practical OSCE examination (set by external, volunteering examiners).

Specialty Certificates

Successful completion of the curriculum results in the award of the title of "Fellow" (post-nominal "FKBMS") by KBMS or the MSc in radiation oncology by the University of Sulaimani.

Part II: Adjunctive Collaborative Opportunities

Internal Academic Assistance

Radiation oncology practice is closely related to many basic and clinical sciences. Based on the syllabus, contact with local academics at the University of Sulaimani was arranged to cover the required subjects. All of them enthusiastically helped in covering the syllabus.

International Individual Assistance

Individual contacts with colleagues in different disciplines and countries were made to arrange short professional visits to ZCC. This proved to be successful. Many colleagues from various disciplines and countries (Jordan, Saudi Arabia, the UK, the USA, Canada, and Italy) visited ZCC and spent days to weeks working voluntarily with the local mentors and residents. These visitors shared their expertise as lecturers and trainers and as external examiners in the final year of OSCE examination for the first cohort in May 2017.

Global Institutional Networking

Considerable efforts were made to establish external outreach with international centers and organizations. Memoranda of understanding were arranged with centers in Turkey, India, the USA, and Canada. ZCC obtained membership of the most extensive global umbrella for cancer control, the Union for International Cancer Control (UICC), making it the first in Iraq.

ACR (American College of Radiology) In-Training Examination

In an endeavor to standardize our training program in line with international programs in developed countries, the American College of Radiology allowed our residents to enroll in its annual in-training examination in March 2017 after arranging the required examination fees. Seven ZCC residents sat the examination on the same day as their peers in the USA. They did well in general; even one of them passed his peers' mean in the USA. This provides benchmarking for both the residents and their program.

This orientation and benchmarking experience was, however, not repeated due to financial hardship of the ZCC resulting in a lack of providing the necessary infrastructure for its proper conduct. It would be desirable to provide this examination for the current and coming residents in order to secure an objective measure for the teaching success.

Scientific Meetings and Courses

To further improve evidence-based, multidisciplinary approaches to cancer care, ZCC was successful in arranging the following four international activities:

- Multi-Disciplinary Oncology Course series in Iraq (February 2015) covered general cancer care, a five-day course attended by 206 attendees.
- Best of ASTRO Iraq meeting (December 2015), officially licensed by ASTRO, covered best abstracts from the 2015 annual ASTRO meeting, with 197 attendees.
- Multi-Disciplinary Oncology Course series in Iraq, second course, covered gynecologic oncology in September 2016, over 2 days, attended by 227 attendees.
- Best of ASTRO Iraq meeting (May 2017), officially licensed by ASTRO, covered best abstracts from the 2016 annual ASTRO meeting, attended by 152 attendees.

In addition to attendance and benefiting from these events' scientific opportunities, the residents presented their work and assumed organizational and leadership roles. The invited external speakers shared their expertise in teaching the residents through dedicated "meet the professor" sessions. They also joined ZCC examination days that were arranged in the periods of the meetings.

Online Education and Telemedicine Tools

Some of the program residents were able to further improve their educational knowledge through accessing ESTRO School FALCON courses (Fellowship in Anatomic DeLineation and CONtouring). One of the residents, who participated in this international course in 2017, came first among all the international participants and was acknowledged by IAEA during the International Conference in Advanced Radiation Oncology in Vienna, June 2017.

Quality and Safety Culture

ZCC fosters a culture of quality and safety. All residents, physicists, therapists, and other staff are obliged to report any incidents or accidents during daily work. An emphasis on the double- and triple-check is the norm to improve patient care safety and quality. This includes but is not limited to contours and plan check, treatment delivery, and the entire patient care process.

External Training Opportunities

Some of the residents participated in a palliative care course organized locally by an international expert. Other residents attended international clinical attachments for some days and weeks to months at advanced centers in Turkey, the UK, and the USA.

Research Promotion and Collaboration

Simultaneously and in parallel with the education and clinical training program, research activities were supported. During the period 2013–2018, ZCC residents and staff accomplished 2 books, 7 theses, 10 peer-reviewed manuscripts, 19 oral presentations (5 were international), and 17 poster international presentations covering miscellaneous topics (Mula-Hussain et al. 2019b). ZCC hosted an international student from the University of Toronto for 4 weeks in 2017 to let her voluntarily help in a supervised medical and laboratory experience and assist in the residents' research activities from the English language editing perspective.

Local Funding and Supporting Opportunities

Civil society, nongovernmental organizations, the private sector, and philanthropic individuals in Sulaimani and across Iraq were approached to help the training center and its educational programs and scientific activities. This proved to be helpful to ZCC in furthering its clinical and educational mission. These opportunities helped in covering the costs of the four scientific events that ZCC arranged, the membership cost at UICC, partial support of the external visits that the residents did abroad, costs of the travel and accommodation expenses of the external short-stay trainers and lecturers, updating some of the tools and equipment at ZCC, etc.

Follow-Up

After beginning the program in 2013, new cancer cases almost doubled compared to 2012. The center's registry reported 1040 in 2013 compared to 655 in 2012. This increased gradually to 1155 in 2015. In addition to the standard baseline three-dimensional conformal radiotherapy, more services started after launching the training program in ZCC, such as intensity-modulated radiation therapy (IMRT) in the mid-2013 and high-dose rate brachytherapy in the mid-2016, both for the first time in Iraq.

To date (2021), ten residents had enrolled and completed its requirements and are currently working independently. Eight of them initially were the local ZCC residents who had enrolled in 2013 and 2014 in two different batches and presently working as specialists in ZCC itself. Another two were from other centers, and they returned to their home centers in Mosul and Erbil (350 km and 200 km from Sulaimani, respectively). The program is still running with four ongoing residents in its path.

Niloy R. Datta et al. reported in 2014 that only 4 of 139 low- and middle-income countries (LMICs) have the requisite number of MVMs and 55 (39.5%) have no radiation oncology facilities (Datta et al. 2014). Patient's access to radiotherapy in the remaining 80 LMICs ranges from 2.3% to 98.8% (median: 36.7%). By 2020, these 84 LMICs would additionally need 12,149 radiation oncology practitioners (Datta et al. 2014).

While currently there is no apparent shortage in radiation oncology workforce at ZCC and Sulaimani as a city, the deficit is evident in the number of machine that is not enough for the governorate itself. The gap will be more pronounced when we know that ZCC accepts patients from any place in Iraq, particularly those who come from the governorates that do not have radiotherapy services. There is a significant shortage of the ideal MVM number and the radiation oncology practitioners in Iraq as a whole country. These gaps will increase in the future due to population growth unless there will be good momentum in advancing the human resources and the functional MVMs. In 2019, in the whole country, there were about 49 radiation oncologists (Ministry of Health/Environment 2019) and 19 MVMs (International Atomic Energy Agency 2020), to serve the 35,864 new cancer patients (Iraqi Cancer Board 2020), among the 39 million Iraqis in 2019–2020. Based on the ratio of one MVM per one million population that can be suitable to Iraq, the coverage in 2019 was about 46% of the ideal MVMs (International Atomic Energy Agency 2008). In 2022, the estimates are 52,855 new cancer cases over 42 million Iraqi population, and this necessitates additional human resources and MVMs to decrease the gap in radiotherapy across the country.

Conclusions

After 18 months of logistical preparation and over 4 years of structured and accredited training in the 2010s, the process of establishing the 4-year board-certified residency program in Iraq was accomplished (2013–2017) (Mula-Hussain et al. 2019a, b). Despite all the challenges, the program continued running till now. This program's success was significantly driven by the high level of enthusiasm of all those involved, including trainees, as well as other personnel from the academics and leaders of the institutions involved. We believe that this successful experience is noteworthy, and it can serve as a model for other developing unstable nations.

Perseverance paid off as it became the first board-certified program in radiation oncology established in Iraq. Ten physicians (including two female colleagues) completed the training requirements in radiation oncology in 2017–2020, seven with the four-year board KBMS program and three with the three-year MSc university program. They are serving six Iraqi governorates (Sulaimani, Erbil, Duhok, Halabja, Kirkuk, and Mosul) with a combined population of over ten million.

ZCC was successful in its vision, and it achieved the mission with its bridging program. ZCC staff are transitioning from being general certified radiation oncology practitioners to being site-specific radiation oncology practitioners. Each specialist is responsible for 2–3 cancer sites to master their expertise further. The program is still running with ongoing residents in its path.

It took a team of local professionals and a global collaboration with medical institutions dedicated to elevating the standard of cancer care to have this success story. We believe that many countries that are similarly coming out of war may achieve similar success. This experience can be duplicated in other underserved developing countries if the minimum requirements are available.

Acknowledgments Many individuals and organizations contributed to the success of this project. The names are too numerous to list here. To all of them, we express our sincere appreciation.

References

Al-Ghazi M (2016) Cancer care in a war zone: radiation oncology in Iraq. Int J Radiat Oncol Biol Phys 96(2, Supplement):E413

Datta NR, Samiei M, Bodis S (2014) Radiation therapy infrastructure and human resources in low- and middle-income countries: present status and projections for 2020. In reply to Sharma et al. Int J Radiat Oncol Biol Phys 90(4):971–972

International Atomic Energy Agency (2008) Setting up a radiotherapy programme: clinical, medical physics, radiation protection and safety aspects, 1st edn. International Atomic Energy Agency - IAEA, Vienna

International Atomic Energy Agency (2009) IAEA syllabus for the education and training of radiation oncologists, Vienna. https://www-pub.iaea.org/MTCD/Publications/PDF/TCS-36_web.pdf

International Atomic Energy Agency (2010) Planning national radiotherapy services : a practical tool. International Atomic Energy Agency, Vienna. http://www-pub.iaea.org/MTCD/Publications/PDF/Pub1462_web.pdf

International Atomic Energy Agency (2017) In: Rosenblatt E, Zubizarreta E (eds) Radiotherapy in Cancer Care: Facing the Global Challenge | IAEA, 1st edn. International Atomic Energy Agency, Vienna. [cited 2020 May 2]. http://www-pub.iaea.org/MTCD/Publications/PDF/P1638_web.pdf

International Atomic Energy Agency (2020) DIRAC (DIrectory of RAdiotherapy Centres). Vol 2018. https://dirac.iaea.org/Query/Countries

Iraqi Cancer Board (2020) Annual Report - Iraqi Cancer Registry 2019. Baghdad; [cited 2021 Feb 18]. https://moh.gov.iq/upload/upfile/ar/1422.pdf

Ministry of Health/Environment (2019) Annual statistical report. Baghdad. [cited 2020 Nov 20]. https://moh.gov.iq/upload/upfile/ar/1090.pdf

Mula-Hussain L (2012) Cancer care in Iraq: a descriptive study, 1st edn. LAP LAMBERT Academic Publishing, Saarbrucken-Germany

Mula-Hussain L (2013) Training handbook of the Kurdistan Board in Radiation Oncology, 1st edn. Kurdistan Board of Medical Specialties, Sulaimani

Mula-Hussain L, Al-Ghazi M (2020) Cancer care in times of war: radiation oncology in Iraq. Int J Radiat Oncol Biol Phys 108(3):523–529

Mula-Hussain L, Shamsaldin A, Younis SN, Mohammad MO, Ramzi ZS, Ahmed ZA et al (2019a) Establishment of 1st board-certified radiation oncology residency program in a war-torn nation: experience from Iraq. Radiother Oncol 139:S84–S85

Mula-Hussain L, Shamsaldin AN, Al-Ghazi M, Muhammad HA, Wadi-Ramahi S, Hanna RK et al (2019b) Board-certified specialty training program in radiation oncology in a war-torn country: challenges, solutions and outcomes. Clin Transl Radiat Oncol 19:46–51. http://www.sciencedirect.com/science/article/pii/S2405630819300904

Mula-Hussain L, Wadi-Ramahi SJ, Zaghloul MS, Al-Ghazi M (2019c) Radiation oncology in the Arab world. In: Laher I (ed) Handbook of healthcare in the Arab world. Springer International Publishing, Cham, pp 1–19. https://doi.org/10.1007/978-3-319-74365-3_151-1

Mula-Hussain L, Wadi-Ramahi S, Li B, Ahmed S, Ynoe De Moraes F (2021) Specialty Portfolio in Radiation Oncology A global certification roadmap for trainers and trainees (Handbook-Logbook). Qatar University Press. [cited 2021 Feb 15]. http://qspace.qu.edu.qa/handle/10576/17692

Zhianawa Cancer Center (2017) Zhianawa Cancer Center. Vol. 2018. http://www.zhianawa.org/

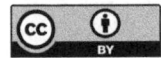

Improving the WHO Classification of Tumours by an Evidence-Based Approach: A New Online/Blended Learning Training Program

Blanca Iciar Indave Ruiz

The *WHO Blue Books*

Diagnosis and classification of individual cancers underpin treatment and care of cancer patients, as well as research into cancer epidemiology, prevention, diagnosis, and treatment. Traditionally, cancer classification has been based on consensus of histopathological opinion, with very limited consideration of more recent aspects as advances in molecular pathology or the use of evidence-based practices to inform decisions. However, new technologies are transforming the field rapidly, and it has become increasingly clear that the traditional approach to cancer classification is insufficient. The understanding of cancer at a molecular level, the advances in prognosis and prediction, as well as the fast development of methods to assess related evidence has now reached a point where this information must be included in the decision-making process of the classification and diagnoses of cancer. Other fields such as digital pathology and image analysis are also producing new insights, challenging many diagnostic criteria and showing an urgent need to integrate these facets of diagnosis into cancer classification internationally using an appropri-ate evidence-based approach. Also, the fast development of related scientific areas as omics or biotechnology has added pressure to the process of assessing the evidence in a timely manner, contributing extensively to the information overload in the field. More than one million papers pour into the PubMed database each year (about two papers per minute) (Landhuis 2016), challenging experts who are already over-whelmed by publishing and other time-eaters.

The International Agency for Research on Cancer (IARC) has been responsible for the *World Health Organization (WHO) Classification of Tumours* since its third edition and is in charge of updating the classification on a regular basis, the fifth edition of this classification currently being under production. Published as the *WHO Blue Books* and the *WHO Blue Books* online (Fig. 1) (*WHO Classification of Tumours* 2019), this is an essential resource for pathologists and cancer researchers worldwide. They provide the standards against which tumors are classified and are key in cancer diagnosis, while also support-ing cancer research, treatment, and prognosis. Each book summarizes the characteristics of one tumor type, including diagnostic criteria, pathological features, and associated molecular altera-tions. One edition covers all organ sites in 14 volumes, describing and illustrating in a strictly disease-oriented manner each single tumor type to provide the international standards for diagno-sis and cancer research.

B. I. I. Ruiz (✉)
WHO Classification of Tumours Group, International Agency for Research on Cancer, Lyon, France
e-mail: IndaveI@iarc.fr

U. Schmidt-Strassburger (ed.), *Improving Oncology Worldwide*, Sustainable Development Goals Series,
https://doi.org/10.1007/978-3-030-96053-7_6

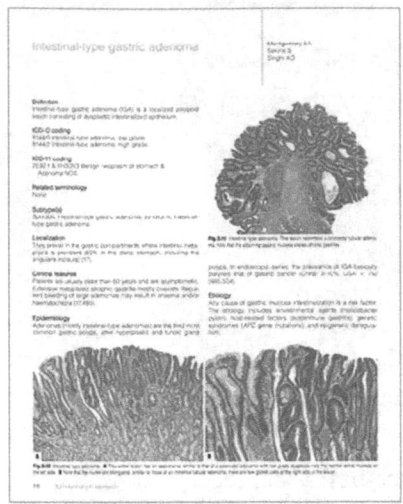
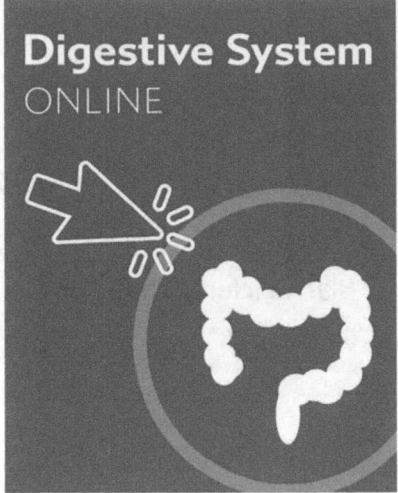
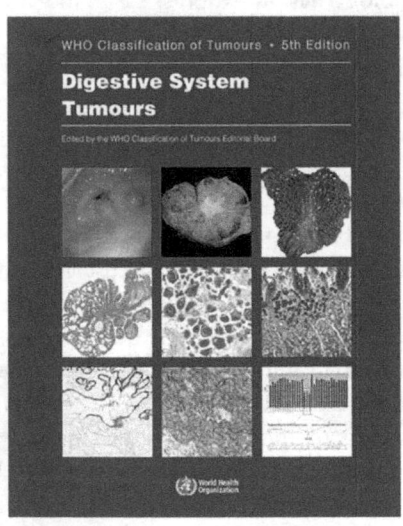

Fig. 1 The *World Health Organization (WHO) Classification of Tumours* (fifth edition), published as the *WHO Blue Books* and the *WHO Blue Books* online

The fifth edition of the *WHO Classification of Tumours (WCT)* contains on average 300 tumor types per book and provides a definition for each type followed by a description of relevant features with the same structure for all. Aspects such as etiology, pathogenesis, epidemiology, clinical features, macroscopic appearances, histology, cytology, molecular pathology, essential and desirable diagnostic features, staging, prognostic factors, and predictive biomarkers are summarized, and all require a review of the scientific literature to assess available evidence. Sometimes conflictive decisions need to be taken, and it is most relevant to inform these decisions with the best available evidence. To retrieve this evidence and to evaluate and summarize it while minimizing the risk of introducing bias, evidence-based practice methods have to be followed, and for this reason, increasingly systematic review methods have been introduced in the processes informing the WCT. But performing systematic reviews for all is not feasible. If each section describing one aspect related to one single tumor type were to require at least one formal review, that would mean conducting more than 3000 reviews for a book, which would not be practicable and highly inefficient. The current approach therefore relies largely on literature searches for published articles performed by the same subject experts that contribute to the books, being based on their individual perceptions of need for the assessment of the content of these books. Yet, these decisions affect the classification and hence the diagnosis and management of cancer patients worldwide. So, to minimize the risk of including biased information, an editorial board composed of standing members and content experts (mainly practicing pathologists) takes the final decisions agreeing in structured meetings on definitions and core criteria for each tumor systematically for every new edition.

Adapting the Current Procedure to Information Overload

Overreliance on expert consensus at editorial board meetings may lead to problems, and IARC undertakes continuous efforts to understand how this may affect the WCT (Table 1). In a recent analytical exercise (Uttley et al. 2020), the WCT group together with international experts identified key elements of the process that need to be taken into account before drafting recommendations for improvement of the evidence base of the classification. They acknowledged the need to review evidence in order to assess all relevant issues in a *WHO Blue Books* but also realized that different expertise and inevitable time constraints of participating experts would result in highly variable results with a potential for studies relevant to decisions to be missed. Not all issues need to be assessed by systematic reviews (Collins and Fauser 2005; Ioannidis 2016), a background search often being sufficient to assess statements not relevant to classification issues. These were also the findings of an informal exploration of the initial *WCT* fifth edition books showing each book to contain over 100 subjects described as "unknown" and more than 200 labelled as "clinically not relevant," often without any additional description of the section or references (*WHO Classification of Tumours* 2019). Also, sections such as etiology and pathogenesis are frequently described as "unknown," yielding uncertainty

whether an exhaustive search of the literature had been performed to affirm the notion. This does not necessarily indicate that systematic reviews should be routinely performed, considering the impracticality to produce the required numbers in time. Many statements are more related to background information provided for the classification of the tumor type and less so to decisions relevant to classification. Insisting on systematic approaches would probably not improve the evidence base of the classification per se, while relying on simple background searches for this type of assessment would give authors the chance to invest more efforts in pressing issues: topics that need to be assessed by systematic reviews due to their potential for controversy.

In the previously mentioned analytical exercise (Uttley et al. 2020), authors discussed also that relying on consensus of the editorial board without a structured and controlled process of evidence synthesis may include unintended bias from content experts and influence decisions. Certain studies could be given more value, overlooked, or misunderstood depending on the clinical or research background of the authors (Young 2009). Authors also pointed out that the representativeness of the expert panel was key to avoid skewed decisions that may not be fully informed by the best and most relevant evidence (Doust and Del Mar 2004; McKee et al. 1991) and that language skills and personal and cultural differences in expert panels may lead to discussions being dominated by individuals (Doust and Del Mar 2004; McKee et al. 1991; Kea and Sun 2015). And lastly, concerns about previous errors in referenced evidence being carried forward during the subsequent updates were discussed.

Controversies Pertaining to Evidence-Based Approaches in Pathology

The WCT has an important influence of incorporating noncommercial knowledge into the diagnosis for patient management, as well as repercussions in clinical diagnosis and management of cancer patients, which is why much effort is invested in providing the most accurate synthe-

Table 1 Problem arising from consensus-based approach and proposed solutions by an evidence-based approach

Problem of a consensus-based approach	Solution by an evidence-based approach	Potential problems not solved by an evidence-based approach
Risk of missing relevant research	Comprehensive searching—which is part of systematic reviewing—may improve identification of important literature A structured, systematic process allows summarizing and evaluating complex information—such as big data or basic research information—provided for molecular pathology	There is a risk of missing research not fitting into the standard study design framework used for systematic reviews Publication bias may not be addressed if only searching published evidence
Selection of the literature may be biased	Systematic reviews require clearly stated inclusion criteria, so cherry-picking of particular studies to prove a particular point is easier to spot In addition, the setting of acceptable evidence levels and assessment of risk of bias of studies avoids the use of inappropriate evidence	Presentation of results may still allow a certain degree of "cherry-picking" when presenting only on selected outcomes (outcome reporting bias)
Interpretation of the literature may be biased	Systematic reviews consider each included study equally, unless there is a specific reason why less emphasis should be placed on it such as small sample or poor study quality Risk of bias assessment of individual studies, but also of the body of evidence, can be undertaken to aid an appropriate interpretation of the retrieved evidence	The use of several reviewers may not provide the desired control of bias effect, and instead interesting information may not be incorporated due to disagreement
Panel of experts may be biased in composition or be dominated by particular individuals	A systematic review with clear eligibility criteria made available in a protocol may provide a reference point against which "extreme" views by particular panel members can be mitigated	Panel may still be biased in developing eligibility criteria, even if an evidence-based approach helps in the discussion
Difficulties in documentation of included evidence (especially in the updating process)	Systematic review protocols and reports document the biomedical databases searched and over what time period. Therefore, uncertainty about whether a particular study has been included or not is much less likely to occur	It relies on the well-designed and appropriate literature searches and implementation of reporting standards for systematic reviews
Credibility of classification may be undermined if not evidence based	The use of systematic review methods will improve the credibility of the classification, as well as the reliability of tumor classification	Credibility may also be affected by other factors not addressed by a systematic review process Experts in the field, important to the credibility of the books, may be put off by the systematic review process

Source: Uttley, L., Indave, B.I., Hyde, C., White, V., Lokuhetty, D. and Cree, I. (2020), Invited commentary—WHO Classification of Tumours: How should tumours be classified? Expert consensus, systematic reviews or both? Int. J. Cancer, 146: 3516–3521. https://doi.org/10.1002/ijc.32975

sis of the scientific evidence to inform all decisions relevant to the international standards which underpin the diagnosis of individual tumor types. To mitigate the previously described problems, a progressive addition of evidence-based practices to the editorial process of the WCT has been planned, as well as the promotion of evidence-based pathology and the performance of systematic reviews in the field to facilitate the rapid incorporation of best available evidence. Systematic reviews are widely regarded as the cornerstone of evidence-based medicine, hence the best available evidence to inform decisions, because they include comprehensive literature searching, transparency in methods, and rigorous evidence appraisal (Higgins 2008; Mulrow 1994).

However, even if performing systematic reviews to assess certain aspects of a tumor type could improve the reliability of decisions taken by the editorial board, important limitations exist to the regular application of such methods. Training in methods and expertise is required to perform well a systematic review (Gotzsche and Ioannidis 2012; Piehl et al. 2003; Uttley and Montgomery 2017), they are laborious, time-consuming, and difficult to interpret, and these difficulties increase with evidence of low grade. Traditional systematic review methods are often rigid, and best practice guidelines such as Cochrane (Higgins 2008) and PRISMA (Moher et al. 2009) yield numbers closely aligned with meta-analytic reviews for medical interventions and methods that are not necessarily appropriate for research in pathology. Also, critique of the traditional hierarchy of evidence-based medicine with systematic reviews at the top has been registered among clinicians and pathologists for oversimplifying complex clinical diagnostical issues (Williams and Garner 2002; Parker 2005; Murad et al. 2016). Indeed, they are subject to influence if not conducted as objectively as any other research, and managing the influence and expertise of team members in a systematic review remains critical to producing reliable and externally valid conclusions (Uttley and Montgomery 2017).

How to Adapt Evidence Synthesis to the Needs of Pathologists?

Although clearly essential for any evidence synthesis in a controversial question, systematic review methods would need to be adapted to the specific needs of the WCT and its editorial process. Timely assessment of the evidence is one of the major problems for WCT, and this is something that traditional, comprehensive systematic reviews struggle to provide. Modern, alternative review methods including mapping, rapid, or scoping reviews could improve the quality of scientific reviews used to inform decisions in the WCT (Dobbins 2017; Khangura et al. 2012; Polisena et al. 2015; Moher et al. 2015), even though they do increase the risk of introducing

bias and errors during the review process and may not always provide the expected results (Dobbins 2017; Khangura et al. 2012; Haby et al. 2016). Therefore, full systematic reviews of the available evidence should be—for the moment—limited to the assessment of research questions that directly affect the classification of tumor or may have major consequences in cancer diagnosis. And a focus on how to solve these challenges for the WCT editorial process is needed.

Additional problems detected during the editorial process are the low number of high-quality evidence synthesis published in the field of pathology and therefore the difficulties for the WCT authors to retrieve ready-to-use high-level evidence to prove their statements. Scientific production in the field of pathology is frequently at the lowest levels of the evidence pyramid, with publications as case reports, case series, or narrative reviews being common. This is well known and has been explained with motives as being performed by clinical "unfunded" faculty members, the predominantly observational nature of a pathologist's work, or that anatomic pathology is subject to "interobserver variation" and has therefore an inherently higher proneness to error. Also, other quality issues are common as meta-analyses in diagnostic pathology showing less compliance with reporting recommendations such as PRISMA (Liu et al. 2017) or an underutilization of this method (Kinzler and Zhang 2015). Nowhere is this more apparent than in the field of molecular pathology, and it is there where most controversial topics arise with research groups suggesting different tumor classifications based on proposed molecular signatures not taking in consideration what type of evidence needs to be generated to prove such a relationship (Baxter 2003; González-Reymúndez and Vázquez 2020; Mamatjan et al. 2017). The issue of using validated methods for WCT is becoming increasingly important due to these rapid advances with more information becoming evident than from histopathological analysis alone as in former years. Systematic review methods may need to be adapted to assess this information, as some steps of a validated systematic review process may not meet current need, but evidence synthesis and evaluations are needed to assess how to incorporate single molecular advances into the WCT. Also, to be able to perform adequate systematic review studies in the field, standardized reporting recommendations such as the Standards for Reporting Diagnostic Accuracy Studies (STARD) (Cohen et al. 2016), Transparent Reporting of a Multivariable Prediction Model for Individual Prognosis or Diagnosis (TRIPOD) (Moons et al. 2015), and other standardized reporting guidance (www.equator.net) have to be followed by original research allowing for pooling and comparison of their results.

Plan of Action

Herein lies the challenge for the WHO Classification of Tumours: to develop a strategy that helps to move future editions acting at multiple levels toward a more evidence-based approach, where experts take decisions well informed by accurate synthesis of the best available evidence. Steps are already being taken to incorporate systematic and adapted review methods into the editorial process without compromising the much-needed expert consensus. The importance of systematic reviews and expert interpretation does not need to be viewed as mutually exclusive. One should not be seen as superior to another, as each represent necessary concepts of analysis and synthesis (Mickenautsch 2010) and evidence-based medicine has always stated that external evidence can inform, but never replace expertise (Sackett 1997). There is also an opportunity to ensure that research and evidence synthesis in the field of pathology and therefore for the WCT are fit for purpose without enforcing rigid guidelines, just addressing identified challenges in a coordinated manner. At the WCT, we propose an approach that is adapted to the needs of the *WHO Blue Books* which starts by requesting contributing authors to employ a series of "nonnegotiables" while performing the literature reviews that feed into key decisions for the classification. Table 2 shows the rationale and risk underlying each proposed "nonnegotiable."

It ends with the provision of training in systematic review methods to a broad spectrum of pathologists, oncologists, and researchers contributing with their work to the body of evidence consulted to classify tumors. Experts, who serve as authors and editors, require basic training on epidemiological essential knowledge to be able to critically appraise their findings and also methodological support in systematic review and literature searching methods that can be provided by the WCT secretariat. Other important challenges for the WCT such as the application of the differing evidence levels and considerations within the field of pathology are addressed by projects initiated by the WCT program, projects that search for consensus in the field to promote a comparable assessment of studies. Furthermore, a register is planned where topics in need for assessment are listed and prioritized based on WCT requirements and scientific considerations.

The IC3R Initiative

IARC and the WCT program have set ourselves the challenge to continuously revise our procedures to keep incorporating evidence-based practices into the current expert-led approach and follow continuous improvement principles for our editorial process. The privileged position of IARC in the field allowed us to initiate a representative international collaboration that joins actions to identify potential challenges and solutions for tumor classification and for cancer research in general: the International Collaboration for Cancer Classification and Research or in short, IC^3R (https://ic3r.iarc.who.int/). This collaboration aims to provide a unique forum for coordinating evidence generation, for synthesis and evaluation, and for tumor classification and cancer research, as well as related issues as standard setting or developing best practice recommendations (Cree et al. 2021). IC^3R facilitates the communication between the WCT editorial board and the multiple scientific communities producing the body of evidence used to inform decisions in the classification

Table 2 Methodological nonnegotiables for systematic reviews for the purposes of tumor classification

Rationale	Risks (if not considered in the review)
1. Transparency	
Methods should be clearly stated and previously defined. Inclusion and exclusion criteria are stated and applied A review protocol should be written and made publicly available as an explicit statement of intended methods where deviations to these methods can be noted (with justifications). This ensures accountability by authors and facilitates replication of the review Conflict of interests of the review team as well as funding information needs to be disclosed	• Methods may not be appropriate to ensure equitable representation of literature globally • Unjustified deviations to planned methods remain unchallenged • Undeclared conflicts of interest or researcher allegiance from authors may influence conclusions
2. Searching rigor	
Searching two major bibliographic databases (e.g., PubMed and web of science) minimizes the chance that a highly relevant study will be missed. While there are overlaps in medical bibliographic databases, indexing varies considerably. Therefore, searching only one database means that retrieval of relevant literature is highly dependent on appropriateness/accuracy of the search strategy	• Reliance on one database capturing all relevant studies, reliance on all relevant studies being accurately indexed, and reliance on a single search strategy being sufficient to capture all relevant literature • Failure to identify all relevant literature
3. Double-checking	
Duplication of the data extraction and a proportion of the total study selection done by the primary author should be completed by a second reviewer for accuracy. Where multiple discrepancies are noted, further checking may be required for consistency	• Reliance on the accuracy and consistency of one author for all study selection and data extraction • Bias in selection of studies • Greater chance of erroneous study selection or data extraction
4. Risk of bias assessment	
A methodological quality assessment tool for pathology reviews should be adapted, based on a standardized risk of bias assessment tool. This helps review authors to assign more weight to findings from studies of higher quality or at lower risk of bias in interpretation	• No objective method of appraising studies for higher risk of bias • Biases from primary studies are perpetuated in the review • Bias in interpretation of studies may be applied by review authors

Source: Uttley, L., Indave, B.I., Hyde, C., White, V., Lokuhetty, D. and Cree, I. (2020), Invited commentary—WHO Classification of Tumours: How should tumours be classified? Expert consensus, systematic reviews or both? Int. J. Cancer, 146: 3516–3521. https://doi.org/10.1002/ijc.32975

(Fig. 2). Member institutions include universities, research centers, and other interested parties that assign representatives to discuss and coordinate international efforts for the provision of concrete deliverables needed to set standards and to underpin the WHO Classification of Tumours and cancer research in general (Fig. 3).

The aims of the collaboration include—among others—the harmonization of cancer-related research; the production of evidence evaluations for clinical settings, cancer research, and epidemiology; the identification of research and information gaps; and the promotion of evidence-based pathology and evidence-based practice in related

fields. All objectives align with evidence-based medicine principles that have already been successfully addressed in other specialized medical fields. For this reason, a project was proposed with the aim to reproduce successful examples of the promotion of evidence-based medicine in a medical field as the Cochrane Collaboration (https://www.cochrane.org/) or the Joanna Briggs Institute (https://jbi.global/).

The evidence-based pathology project of IC³R (Cree et al. 2021) is the first project to be initiated under the framework of the collaboration and addresses the challenges of producing an evidence-based tumor classification, including

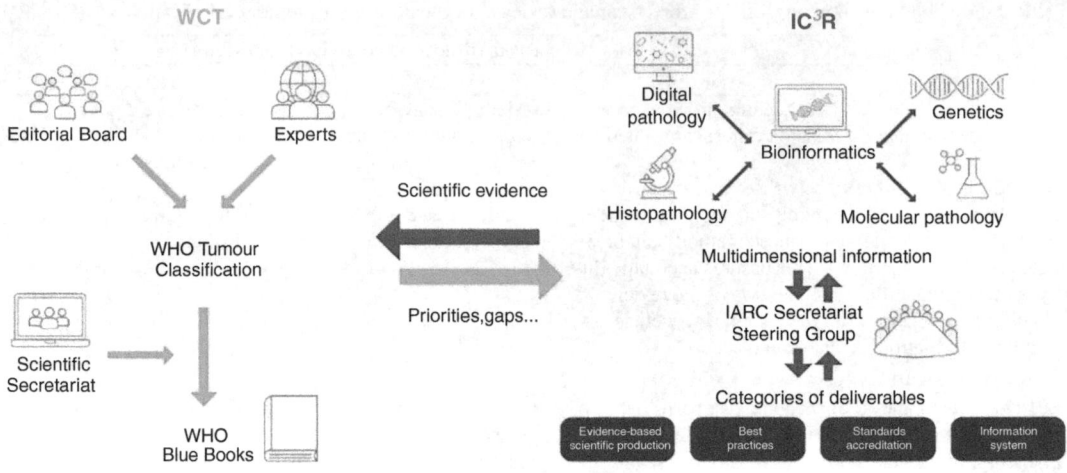

Fig. 2 Framework of the International Collaboration for Cancer Classification and Research (IC³R)

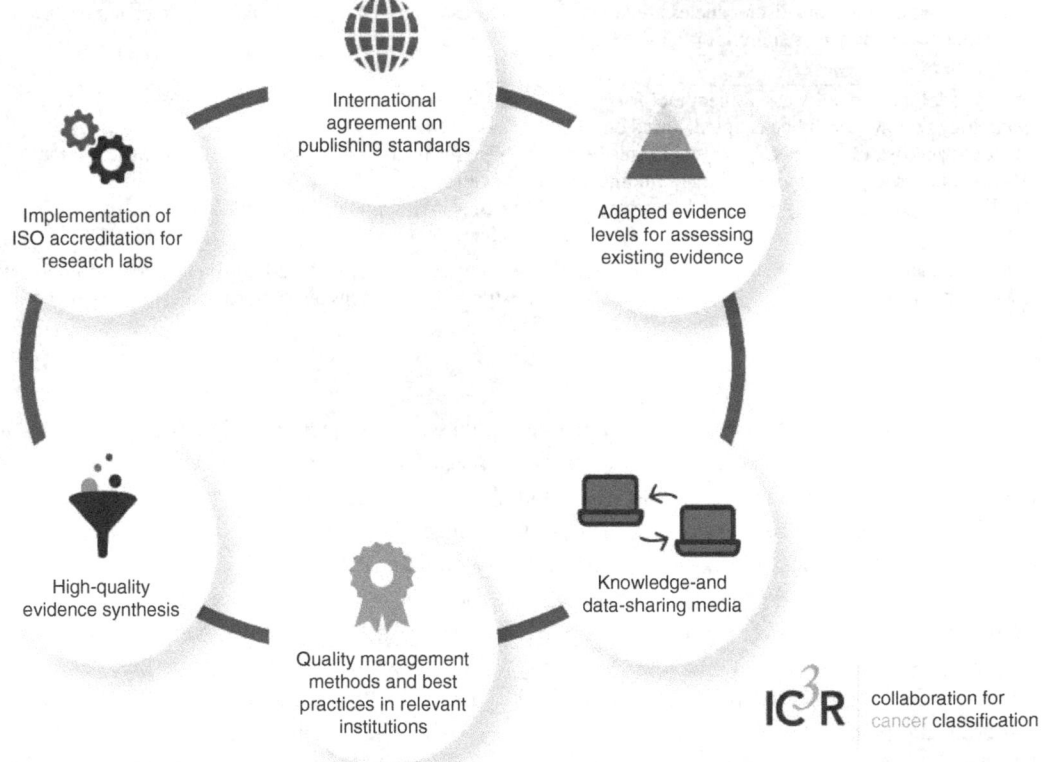

Fig. 3 Expected impact of the International Collaboration for Cancer Classification and Research (IC3R)

deliverables such as adapted evidence levels for the field, new systematic review methods, training in evidence-based pathology, systematic review tools, and the development of a network of reviewers and supervisors to further develop and spread evidence-based pathology. Such an evidence-based pathology movement, with sufficient resources and adequate coordination, could respond with evidence-based assessments to the predicted large number of decisions that will have to be addressed for tumor classification. And IC³R is ideally positioned to efficiently promote and coordinate such an endeavor, working with other partners in pathology and drawing on the expertise of the more widespread evidence-based movements. The project is planned as a multiple partner joint action, where partners such as the University of Ulm (Germany), the Cochrane Centre (Netherlands), and the Exeter Test Group of the University of Exeter (United Kingdom) contribute to different work packages with their distinct expertise. At the beginning, the focus will be on the design of new methodologies and the development of a training program for experts, to allow the construction of an extended network of evidence-based pathology hubs in subsequent phases.

Evi-Pat

The Evidence-Based Pathology Training Initiative (Evi-Pat) started working on the development of a new training program for this purpose in the summer of 2020 and developed a proposal for a new online training in evidence-based practice and systematic review methods especially developed for pathologists, oncologists, and experts in the field of cancer. This training focuses on adapting methods to the type of evidence used and produced in cancer-related practice and in teaching systematic review methods to experts in the field. Overcoming reluctance to the application of evidence-based medicine (EBM) principles and promoting the development of an evidence-based pathology movement among early career professionals in the field are

further objectives of Evi-Pat. The collaborators are jointly developing a research project to design and produce this educational tool adapted to the times of COVID-19 restrictions with virtual and in-person elements and to compare its performance to an online-only experience in terms of knowledge transfer and user satisfaction. Also, the added value of such an adapted training program for pathology and oncology is meant to be evaluated, as well as the delivery of the module to pathologists and experts from the field of oncology.

This module will be the first deliverable of the work package on training from the evidence-based pathology project and will support effective teaching, research, and networking on evidence-based pathology and oncology for professionals in a manner that is resourceful and—hopefully—applicable in every place in the world with an Internet connection. Outcomes of the full research project will be used to develop a full evidence-based pathology training program over time and help to promote principles of evidence-based medicine in the field of pathology and oncology to better inform decisions of the WCT. Examples such as the Cochrane Collaboration (https://www.cochrane.org/) and the Campbell Collaboration (https://www.campbellcollaboration.org/) have already shown that a collaborative effort can improve the evidence base of decision-making in a whole field, and drawing on the expertise of the more widespread evidence-based movements is one of the impacts of promising predictors of this project.

Conclusion

We believe that an evidence-based approach to informing key decisions that feed into tumor classification will allow the WCT editorial board to mitigate the potential inclusion of biased decisions into the classification and also benefit authors by providing structured, transparent, and reliable methods for the synthesis of available evidence for each tumor type, as the same time as training to apply these methodologies. Our hope over time is that this approach will increase the rigor of the decisions feeding into WCT, by addressing critical questions and identifying research gaps, as well as reaching recommendations for research to inform future editions. Such an approach will maintain the reliability of tumor classification and help to provide solutions to challenges like the exponential rise in number of scientific publications and the need to manage new types of information such as evidence from genetics or big data.DisclaimerThe content of this article represents the personal views of the authors and does not represent the views of the authors' employers and associated institutions. Where authors are identified as personnel of the International Agency for Research on Cancer/ World Health Organization, the authors alone are responsible for the views expressed in this article, and they do not necessarily represent the decisions, policy, or views of the International Agency for Research on Cancer/World Health Organization.

References

Baxter C (2003) Molecular signatures. Nat Rev Genet 4(2):84

Cohen JF, Korevaar DA, Altman DG, Bruns DE, Gatsonis CA, Hooft L et al (2016) STARD 2015 guidelines for reporting diagnostic accuracy studies: explanation and elaboration. BMJ Open 6(11):e012799

Collins JA, Fauser BC (2005) Balancing the strengths of systematic and narrative reviews. Hum Reprod Update 11(2):103–104

Cree IA, Indave Ruiz BI, Zavadil J, McKay J, Olivier M, Kozlakidis Z et al (2021) The international collaboration for cancer classification and research. Int J Cancer 148(3):560–571

Dobbins M (2017) Rapid review guidebook. Steps for conducting a rapid review. [Guideline]. The National Collaborating Centre of Methods and Tools (NCCMT), Canada. https://www.nccmt.ca/uploads/media/media/0001/01/a816af720e4d587e13d-a6bb307df8c907a5dff9a.pdf

Doust J, Del Mar C (2004) Why do doctors use treatments that do not work? BMJ 328(7438):474–475

González-Reymúndez A, Vázquez AI (2020) Multi-omic signatures identify pan-cancer classes of tumors beyond tissue of origin. Sci Rep 10(1):8341

Gotzsche PC, Ioannidis JP (2012) Content area experts as authors: helpful or harmful for systematic reviews and meta-analyses? BMJ 345:e7031

Haby MM, Chapman E, Clark R, Barreto J, Reveiz L, Lavis JN (2016) What are the best methodologies for rapid reviews of the research evidence for evidence-informed decision making in health policy and practice: a rapid review. Health Res Policy Syst 14(1):83

Higgins JPGS (2008) Cochrane handbook for systematic reviews of interventions. West Sussex PO19 8SQ. The Cochrane Collaboration and John Wiley & Sons Ltd, Chichester

Ioannidis JP (2016) The mass production of redundant, misleading, and conflicted systematic reviews and meta-analyses. Milbank Q 94(3):485–514

Kea B, Sun BC (2015) Consensus development for healthcare professionals. Intern Emerg Med 10(3):373–383

Khangura S, Konnyu K, Cushman R, Grimshaw J, Moher D (2012) Evidence summaries: the evolution of a rapid review approach. Syst Rev 1:10

Kinzler M, Zhang L (2015) Underutilization of meta-analysis in diagnostic pathology. Arch Pathol Lab Med 139(10):1302–1307

Landhuis E (2016) Scientific literature: information overload. Nature 535(7612):457–458

Liu X, Kinzler M, Yuan J, He G, Zhang L (2017) Low reporting quality of the meta-analyses in diagnostic pathology. Arch Pathol Lab Med 141(3):423–430

Mamatjan Y, Agnihotri S, Goldenberg A, Tonge P, Mansouri S, Zadeh G et al (2017) Molecular signatures for tumor classification: an analysis of the cancer genome atlas data. J Mol Diagn 19(6):881–891

McKee M, Priest P, Ginzler M, Black N (1991) How representative are members of expert panels? Q Assur Health Care 3(2):89–94

Mickenautsch S (2010) Systematic reviews, systematic error and the acquisition of clinical knowledge. BMC Med Res Methodol 10:53

Moher D, Liberati A, Tetzlaff J, Altman DG (2009) Preferred reporting items for systematic reviews and meta-analyses: the PRISMA statement. PLoS Med 6(7):e1000097

Moher D, Stewart L, Shekelle P (2015) All in the family: systematic reviews, rapid reviews, scoping reviews, realist reviews, and more. Syst Rev 4(1):183

Moons KG, Altman DG, Reitsma JB, Ioannidis JP, Macaskill P, Steyerberg EW et al (2015) Transparent reporting of a multivariable prediction model for individual prognosis or diagnosis (TRIPOD): explanation and elaboration. Ann Intern Med 162(1):W1–W73

Mulrow CD (1994) Rationale for systematic reviews. BMJ 309(6954):597–599

Murad MH, Asi N, Alsawas M, Alahdab F. New evidence pyramid Evid Based Med 2016;21(4):125

Parker M (2005) False dichotomies: EBM, clinical freedom, and the art of medicine. Med Humanit 31(1):23–30

Piehl JH, Green S, McDonald S (2003) Converting systematic reviews to Cochrane format: a cross-sectional survey of Australian authors of systematic reviews. BMC Health Serv Res 3(1):2

Polisena J, Garritty C, Umscheid CA, Kamel C, Samra K, Smith J et al (2015) Rapid review summit: an overview and initiation of a research agenda. Syst Rev 4:111

Sackett DL (1997) Evidence-based medicine. Semin Perinatol 21(1):3–5

Uttley L, Montgomery P (2017) The influence of the team in conducting a systematic review. Syst Rev 6(1): 149

Uttley L, Indave BI, Hyde C, White V, Lokuhetty D, Cree I (2020) Invited commentar™ WHO classification of Tumours: how should tumors be classified? Expert consensus, systematic reviews or both? Int J Cancer 146:3516–3521

WHO Classification of Tumours (2019) Digestive system tumours, 5th edn. Lyon: IARC Publications

Williams DD, Garner J (2002) The case against "the evidence": a different perspective on evidence-based medicine. Br J Psychiatry 180:8–12

Young SN (2009) Bias in the research literature and conflict of interest: an issue for publishers, editors, reviewers and authors, and it is not just about the money. J Psychiatry Neurosci 34(6):412–417

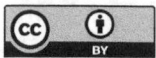

Improving Clinical Research

Andre A. J. Gemeinder de Moraes

Introduction

The Master Online Advanced Oncology Study Program celebrated its tenth anniversary of foundation with a virtual meeting gathering many of the alumni that took part on this recognized initiative from Ulm University.

The program offers an opportunity for professionals involved with research, treatment, and development in the field of oncology, from different countries around the world, to go throughout a period of 2 years of intense study covering all the most important and updated knowledge in the science of oncology, from the basic to applied ones, in a very well-balanced mix of classes online and in attendance. The program brings also the open field for culture exchange among the students, and the unequaled opportunity for an international networking, a fertile field for collaboration.

During the tenth anniversary's virtual meeting, the alumni's community could share their own professional experiences and efforts to accomplish tasks they initiated in their countries. Many experiences were presented, covering educational issues, clinical research, and patient care and also discussing the major challenges in different sites to start institutions devoted to cancer patient care.

In this chapter, we discuss the challenge of clinical research in a broad variety of points of view. The challenge of the discovery of new techniques, new approaches, and mainly new treatments for different kinds of cancers is one of the most critical challenges in clinical research. Different countries and their epidemiological and sanitary needs, and also economic aspects, are very diverse around the world, and these characteristics change the scenarios very much when the researchers seek for answers for their main questions.

Alongside the important questions comes the up-to-date science and international treatment guidelines and recommendations that are not always available in different countries and require smarter initiatives from the local professionals in order to drive the optimal cancer care, available in their countries. We saw this diversity very clearly in the virtual meeting.

Colleagues from everywhere showed how they do research, with different resources and financial support, covering epidemiological data mining, lab research in low-income countries, communication of scientific data, application of advanced molecular and cellular techniques to improve cancer treatment, and challenges to build a clinical research center in an academic environment.

A. A. J. Gemeinder de Moraes (✉)
Clinical Research Unity, Centro de Oncologia
Campinas, Campinas, SP, Brazil

© The Author(s) 2022

U. Schmidt-Strassburger (ed.), *Improving Oncology Worldwide*, Sustainable Development Goals Series,
https://doi.org/10.1007/978-3-030-96053-7_7

As the reader can see, this offers a variety of aspects involved with clinical research and its improvement.

The Different Contributions on Improving Oncology Research

Ahmed Alfaar, MD, working at the Universitätsmedizin Berlin—experimental ophthalmology—shows his experience using data from cancer registries and how these registries can help clinical research. In studying registries, we can generate new hypotheses and take a deep look into epidemiological aspects of different types of cancer and how their outcomes are across different periods of time.

Cancer registries are the cornerstones to the epidemiology of cancer in a population, impacting health-care investments and public health support, and are one of the most important tools to build good plans and right actions to improve the outcome in different health issues.

Dr. Alfaar tells us his experience initiating a cancer registry in Egypt more than a decade ago, pointing out the most challenging issues and their solutions and the improvements following the initiative observed in many aspects of the clinical–research in his institution.

The next chapter of this section brings the experience of Dr. Velizar Shivarov from the Department of Genetics of the Faculty of Biology at the Saint Kliment Ohridski Sofia University—Sofia, Bulgaria—discussing aspects of his experience on data mining as a research option in low- and middle-income countries, other rich life experiences with deep training in different countries, getting back to Sofia and keeping his interest in developing high-level science, and facing a variety of difficulties, but overcoming them with creativity and persistence.

Dr. Carlos Castañeda Altamirano, from the Medical Oncology Department at the Instituto Nacional de Enfermedades Neoplasicas (National Institute of Cancer Maladies), Lima, Peru, describes the need of incorporation of new technologies into the clinical practice treating patients with breast cancer in Peru, based on the multinational clinical research achievements observed when molecular and cellular analysis of breast cancer tissue is performed, with great improvement in the outcome. He discusses important aspects of recent technologies and the importance of its incorporation into the daily practice.

In the final chapter of this section, we can read about the challenges of planning and establishing a Clinical Trials Center, discussed by Dr. Nicole Lang, who is the director of this unit at Ulm University. Efforts are exerted to accomplish many different steps of complexity in order to be compliant with the international and national requirements and regulations and protection of the research subjects, from the protection of data and IT systems, ICH GCP (International Council of Harmonization Good Clinical Practice), to the reliability of the trials' results.

Conclusion

At the end of the tenth anniversary alumni's virtual meeting of the Master Online Advanced Oncology Study Program, a variety of issues and contributions coming from different parts of the world reaffirm the original purposes of the Master's Program offering a wide but detailed view of science in oncology besides a cultural exchange and also a perfect environment to establish a valuable professional network.

After all, the most important message we could learn was that bright minds can do research anywhere in the world. Even a sole person can have an incredible output.

Getting Started in Research: What Registries Can Do for You

Ahmad Samir Alfaar

What Is Research?

Research is a process of questioning paradigms, setting new hypotheses, and challenging the validity of such hypotheses through the proposition of theories that may or may not stand the rigor of scientific testing. This process should result in the development of new knowledge that would be used for the best for humanity. With such new knowledge, novel sets of questions should emerge, leading to further research. In general, the research aims to open new frontiers for the better good of humanity, allowing humankind to expand the boundaries of what is possible and attainable.

From what has been described above, it should become evident that research is a cyclical process. Indeed, research invariably starts with one core idea or set of ideas. Such goals need then to be divided into smaller "achievable" ones. This is followed by a process of prioritizing these ideas and putting them in a logical order, thus creating a research plan. With this plan, a researcher can start working on collecting the data and conducting experiments. Research does not come with-

out its—often considerable—costs. Costs of research stem from the complexity of some research ideas; the need for materials and other experiment-related prerequisites, including human resources, chemicals, travel costs, tools, and space allocation; and in addition the possibility of payments made to patients involved in clinical trials. Funding can be applied for and attained through the potential beneficiaries of research outcomes. Those include private companies that might market and sell a product of research, universities that can benefit from licensing resultant intellectual property, or societies that try to understand the priorities of the research in the community. Applications for funds are often conducted within the context of a call for a grant application or, less frequently, are unsolicited. There are other mechanisms for funding research that can be more complicated, involve multistage revisions, and involve multiple partners/consortia. In these cases, the money granting body usually undergoes ever more complex procedures the more the financial coverage requested. The granting body usually challenges grant applications with multiple tests to affirm the applicability of the research project and ensure that the applicants can accomplish what they claim to be able to do.

Most evaluating committees look at the research idea, its validity, and its logical order in relation to the previously proven facts. This stands at the core of the process of grant applica-

A. S. Alfaar (✉)
Experimental Ophthalmology, Charité—Universitätsmedizin Berlin, Berlin, Berlin, Germany

Department of Ophthalmology, University Hospital of Giessen and Marburg, Giessen, Germany
e-mail: ahmed.alfaar@charite.de

© The Author(s) 2022
U. Schmidt-Strassburger (ed.), *Improving Oncology Worldwide*, Sustainable Development Goals Series,
https://doi.org/10.1007/978-3-030-96053-7_8

tion reviews. When evaluating committees affirm the logic of the research idea, they follow this by evaluating the methods used in conducting the proposed research project. They usually investigate the suitability of the techniques for the intended experimentations and the potential validity of data collected using such techniques. Besides, statistical methods proposed for data analysis are reviewed. Importantly, reviewers also examine how researchers had calculated the required sample size of the patients or participants. Erroneous calculation of sample size has important ethical repercussions, in addition to its effect on the validity of research results. Underestimating the required number of participants would expose humans or animals to potential harm without any statistical value. Likewise, an overestimation of the number of required participants would expose a needless number of patients or lives to potential harm when the hypothesis could have been proven or negated with a lesser number of patients.

Evaluation of the research plan could also involve team structure and their qualifications in relation to the proposed research tasks, as well as the ability of each research sub-team to achieve work packages (a term used for parts of a plan). Individual team members are evaluated separately in terms of their previous achievements. Next, the entire team's work history is examined. A multidisciplinary team—or consortium—with a track record of previous successes would thus more likely win funding for their research proposal. In particular, any successful previous work that is relevant to the proposed research project would play an essential role in a team's successful application.

The evaluation process typically also involves the assessment of the proposed marketing, dissemination, and application of research outcomes. Presentations by researchers should thus include how they had previously conducted marketing and dissemination of their research outcomes as well as their methods of evaluating such processes.

At the start of their careers, most new researchers initially take part in well-funded research projects at well-established research facilities. As they contemplate potentially moving to independent research, they question how these well-funded projects had received funding. While not easy to summarize, we hope that this chapter would shed light on how a new researcher, especially in the epidemiology field, could prepare for the moment when they decide to move to independent research.

What Is a Cancer Registry?

As the name suggests, a cancer registry is a record-keeping method of data pertaining to patients with different cancers. The scope of such a registry could involve data collected at a hospital or a clinic or a group of them. Registries may also collect data pertaining to a small population within a county or a state or bigger populations, that of an entire country or group of countries. Moreover, efforts are conducted by a registry in order to collect data pertaining to the global burden of various cancers. Often, the smaller population cancer registries report to the wider scope ones (Menck and Smart 1994; Jensen et al. 1991).

Typically, efforts to collect information about cancer are conducted for purposes of estimating the burden of disease and making decisions with regard to disease management and resource allocation; countries look at collecting a basic set of information about cancers. Proper data collection requires follow-up and quality assurance, and each collected item necessitates multiple checks and verifications that may compel multiple sources of data. Therefore, most cancer registries prefer to start with a small set of variables and expand with time and advancement of their collection methodologies (Parkin 2006).

There is no single agreed list of data items that should be collected in a cancer registry. However, online resources can help to initiate and decide the scope of a new cancer registry (The International Agency for Research on Cancer (IARC) n.d.). Most cancer registries collect the patients' identifiers to follow up with such patients in the future (if follow-up is included) and to avoid duplication of entries. Other items typically collected include tumor morphology and topography, age at diagnosis, and survival data. The scope of data collected may often be expanded if agreed to between the data collection counterparts. Those counterparts may involve clinics/practices, laboratories, and hospitals. Data collection processes are sometimes enforced by law in order to guarantee a national level of data collection; however, such enforcement does not guarantee the quality of the process and, hence, the resulting outcomes.

For purposes of knowing the burden and trials to disease surveillance, management, and resource allocation, the countries look at collecting a basic set of information about cancers. Due to the required endeavors for data collection, follow-up, and quality assurance, each collected item requires multiple checks and verifications that may necessitate multiple data sources. Historically, most cancer registries preferred to start with a small set of variables and expand with time and advancement of the collection methodologies. Expansion requires additional training of those involved in data collection, especially with large cancer registries where multiple data collection agencies or registrars have to agree on the definitions of the items collected and the milestones of collection and reporting.

After data collection and validation, registries typically report such data both internally and externally. The process of handling data has to be conducted in accordance with internationally agreed ethical norms. The identity of patients involved should always be protected when data is reported.

Security and Privacy

The scope of data collected typically evolves as the aims of a cancer registry change or expand. Commonly, data collected include demographic data, details pertaining to the tumor(s), and data pertaining to survival. Less commonly, data collected may include details of treatment. After some time, a cancer registry may decide to help determine the environmental drivers or psychosocial confounders involved in the burden of a malignancy. Other data collected may include biomolecular or genetic data about the malignan-

cies. Cancer registries may facilitate the integration with other population databases, including health insurance claims and socioeconomic details through national identifiers.

Although this data may represent a wealth of information, it also represents a responsibility to protect the identity of patients/participants. Many studies have shown that such information, which may be minimal in some cases, could still be used to be tracked down to patients, especially those with rare diseases and with the introduction of genomic medicine. Therefore, a debate has arisen regarding whether there should be any widening of the scopes of such registries.

For the aim of fostering scientific ingenuity and research, cancer registries should be able to provide limited access to various data, with levels of clearances/guarantees of anonymity of patients for different "levels" of data provided without hindering scientific progress and innovation. Setting the rules for the data access levels and the minimum reportable groups of patients should be based on further modeling studies that are conducted to examine the datasets (Terry 2012; Hofferkamp 2008). Recent trials are being initiated to use technologies like blockchain to enhance security while connecting multiple data sources (Glicksberg et al. 2020).

Using Registry Data for Research

Although the long introduction I gave may look irrelevant, cancer registries support each of the mentioned aspects. Registry data can provide a base for hypothesis generation and testing for epidemiologic studies. Studies conducted may involve describing specific groups or investigating hypotheses against data collected from a particular population or setting. Through its time and population coverage, it may allow finding incidence and survival differences between groups in addition to temporal and spatial variations (Armstrong 1992; Kumar et al. 2020). Such findings can be correlated with other data from other sources, allowing researchers to detect correlations between cancer incidences and environmental as well as occupational factors. Moreover, such data allow for the comparative assessment of the quality of healthcare services and treatment outcomes between regions and time periods. Furthermore, it can help develop models for the prediction of the impact of diseases, probably on the different socioeconomic slices in the population. Limitless projects can be achieved under the abovementioned paradigms.

For a researcher, it enriches and strengthens their profile in the studied subjects. For grant applicants, working on relevant cancer registry projects together with their future collaborators can provide proof that the proposers can create a functioning team. Besides, working with real-life data adds new skills and statistical challenges to the team and helps for sample size calculations for future studies.

It could allow the team to validate the concepts that are found computationally, for example, if a molecular finding is recorded in a cancer registry, and then the predictive and prognostic significance can be assessed between groups.

The Limitations of Cancer Registries

Cancer registries provide a snapshot or snapshots of patient status at a certain point or multiple points in time. Records do not typically provide a view of patient status or beyond the end of treatment. Multiple treatment milestones could be missed. Therefore, data collected from cancer registries should be analyzed with consideration of the aims and methods used in that registry (Izquierdo and Schoenbach 2000).

Cancer registries vary in their methods of data collection and confirmation, in part due to the nature of their active counterparts. Confirmation of disease in some registries can be based solely upon clinical findings without histopathological confirmation. In other situations, confirmation of data may be based on death certificates only (DCO) which do not typically provide sufficient information about dates of diagnoses or the sites or morphologies of tumors. Such DCO data should be analyzed with caution. The feeding of cancer registries from multiple sources, including hospitals, clinics, pathologists, laboratories,

insurance companies, and death registries, results in a verifiable multidimensional and time-oriented picture of the patients' experience with the disease. Differences in quality/amount of data collected by cancer registries could also be caused by differences in lengths of time chosen for data collection as well as the version of staging or classification system chosen.

Cancer registries that cover geographically dispersed regions face possible discrepancies in training or resources and hence in the quality of the data collection. Cancer registries try to eliminate such discrepancies through training, reporting, policies, and infrastructure standardization.

As I have mentioned, the aims of cancer registries could be different from one to another. As also mentioned, collection milestones could be different, too. Therefore, it is sometimes challenging to aggregate data from different registries, especially when specific questions are being addressed.

The Use of Data from a Cancer Registry Data: One Researcher's Story

Between 2010 and 2014, I worked on initializing a clinical research training program for undergraduates and early graduates at the Children's Cancer Hospital—Egypt 57,357 (Amgad and AlFaar 2014). In that program, I included methods of designing case report forms, data collection, analysis, and reporting. Due to the amount of time it would take for typical data collection and "cleaning," I decided to teach some trainees how to analyze cancer registry data using the Surveillance, Epidemiology, and End Results Program of the US National Cancer Institute (SEER) program instead. The SEER program had been mentioned a few months earlier in the master's program of the Advanced Oncology at Ulm, Germany. Its importance had also been emphasized by our colleague, Mohamed Sabry, the head of the research informatics unit. We, therefore, thought it would be a good candidate to start with SEER as the first topic of the training program. Our student and later colleague, Waleed

Magdy, started investigating the structure of a particular set of data and conducted an analysis of this data (which, at that time, was download-able data). He returned with his first report 2 weeks later. The question I had chosen for him to study was a familiar explorative question from the field of ophthalmic oncology regarding the relative incidence and temporal and spatial patterns of orbital malignancies in the USA. At that time, we had downloaded large data files that we later had to go through and select relevant information. Now SEER data can be accessed through the SEER*Stat Program, which is convenient for those with stable Internet connections, especially when it comes to big queries. In the resultant publication following Sabry's work, we were able to report the incidence of orbital and adnexal tumors and time trends over the years. We reported finding a steady increase in the incidence of lymphomas till the early 2000s (Hassan et al. 2016). We then decided to compare survival data in order to find any potential differences in the survival between orbital tumors in general and orbital lymphomas in particular, as well as potential differences influenced by age (Hassan et al. 2014). Taking this question to the extreme side, Dr. Ibrahim Qaddoumi from St. Jude's Hospital (Memphis, Tennesse, USA) suggested that we focus on the patients that had been afflicted with malignancies in the neonatal period (Alfaar et al. 2017a). Such tumors most probably develop during the intrauterine period. In addition to differences in the distribution of tumors attributed to genetic causes, we found that patients with neonatal tumors had worse survival rates than older ones. This inferior survival had not improved since 1973, despite developments in diagnostic and therapeutic methods. It is noteworthy to say that this detailed collecting of age-specific data required a special "agreement" before using the SEER program. Moreover, we highlighted the major non-oncological causes of death in those patients.

After a discussion with my colleague, Anas Saad, he decided to focus on the topic of non-cancer causes of death in cancer patients. He started investigating possible causes of death in different malignancies. His results shed light on aspects of cancer patient mortality that were previously unknown. We worked together to study the psychological effects of a tumor diagnosis on patients as well as the effects of tumor type and the timing after the diagnosis (Saad et al. 2018). In this study, we have found that in the early diagnosis time and without waiting for any treatment results, there was a significant increase in the suicide rate. We recommended that patients with cancers with known unfavorable progress (such as pancreatic and lung cancers) be given special psychosocial attention and support in the first 3 months after diagnosis. Our investigation of events after cancer diagnosis led us to study the association of cancer diagnoses when multiple malignancies were diagnosed at temporally distant points, as highlighted in previous studies (Harbour et al. 2010). This resulted in finding that pathways involved in the development of uveal melanoma may be shared with other malignancies that were not thought to involve such a pathway before. In the same study, we found an increased incidence of primary systemic tumors following an earlier diagnosis of uveal melanoma (but not the reverse). We attributed this to efforts by oncologists to search for possible metastases following a diagnosis of uveal melanoma. Such efforts would not be conducted to search the uvea for metastases after a diagnosis of malignancies elsewhere in the body (Alfaar et al. 2020).

Another innovation that is soon to come to widespread use is the recruitment of artificial intelligence/machine learning methods to aid in the classification of registry data, especially data that are hard to analyze with conventional techniques.

During that time, we had been developing our hospital-based cancer registry. Our aim was to automate procedures and create routines that update records to overcome the delays imposed by the manual data collection, cleaning, and verification. We were also able to develop routines (or automated verification methods) to check if data had been validated by a set of preset rules. These rules were mainly meant to help clinical practice and to avoid protocol violations. However, we discovered that such routines had also helped the research process by finding anomalies that could not have been discovered by practitioners, including a list of rare presentations or combinations of presentations that had rarely previously been discussed in the literature (Zekri et al. 2015). Having our own database allowed us to learn how to judge other databases. Moreover, it allowed us to link our database with other databases, aggregating data and allowing for better decision-making with regard to local and countrywide issues. We have also tried to overcome the drawbacks of other databases. Furthermore, our registry provided a core of data upon which we started to advance our biorepository and epidemiologic studies (Labib et al. 2016). Based on these achievements, we were able to apply for further research grants and joint collaborations. This proves that establishing a cancer registry is not an end of a story; it draws a path for further research into bettering patient outcomes.

Starting Your Own Registry in a Nutshell

Fourteen years ago, there were only patients, limited resources, a dream of a children's cancer hospital, and determined efforts to fund such a hospital through charity. The founders recruited engineers to build and run the hospital infrastructure and physicians to design, provide, and follow up on treatment plans. However, it was clear that the system required a parallel team that would dig deep in data to provide the evidence for better treatment plans, support the design of measurable protocols, and help follow up the patients closely in conjunction with physicians and pharmacists. The founders decided to establish a research department with the core idea of providing measurement tools that would help improve clinical care. It was destined to be the classic research department that one would find in other countries (Alfaar et al. 2017b). The key to the initiation of this department was a saying by Peter Drucker, who stated that "You cannot manage what you cannot measure." The initial team consisted of eight pharmacists and physicians who were given the title of clinical research associates (CRAs) and clinical research specialists (CRSs). Each of

them was assigned with a group of diseases. They started collecting resources and studying required data and treatment protocols and related studies for the disease they were assigned. Physicians used to write their findings on papers that were gathered in sectioned folders. Folders were kept in central drawers and called once the patient was present in the clinic and archived if the patient died or was lost to follow-up. During study team meetings for each disease, the team discussed different clinical and research topics. The CRAs and CRSs translated these topics into fields in the case report forms. First, the case report forms were disseminated as paper forms and data tabulated in Microsoft Excel sheets. Physicians found it difficult to complete these forms, and data were liable to be lost. Excel sheets were found to be liable to inconsistencies and required extensive cleaning. Later, repeated orientations were conducted for physicians and nurses to stress on the importance of accurate filling of the forms. Excel sheets were converted into MS Access databases which were easier to clean and allowed for some networking. However, with the recruitment of an increasing number of CRAs/CRSs, it became clear that a more network-friendly solution was needed. Therefore, a solution based on MySQL database and PHP programming language provided more networking functions, faster data entry, and cleaner exports. Later, further challenges faced the research teams, including patients developing multiple cancers and study teams requiring multiple changes or modifications of the case report forms. The epidemiology team concomitantly developed multiple survey-based studies and started designing the biobank that required integration with the central patients' records. Therefore, we started looking for a modular and flexible solution to facilitate the integration between projects and keep running while modifications were being made or data are being exported. At that point, hospital management decided to acquire an electronic medical record system. The options for the solution were filtered down to CaBIG and REDCap. The cancer Biomedical Informatics Grid (CaBIG), which NCI provided, was a good candidate because we decided to use the CaTissue solution for managing biobanking which is made by NCI to be easily integrated with CaBIG (Whippen et al. 2007). However, The REDCap solution from the University of Vanderbilt was chosen to manage the research data space because of its more straightforward setup and maintenance (Harris et al. 2009). In parallel, we developed a solution for importing data from EMR to REDCap and another one based on R, R-Shiny, and PHP that would connect with REDCap and develop data aggregates, statistics, and graphs in real time. This required developing and refining previously specified data management and analysis plans and defining data release and transfer policies. The need for these changes became pressing in order to integrate with the then-emerging national cancer registry program.

The final program resulted in a path where the initial patients' data are typed into the electronic medical records as the patient registers in the hospital. These data are transferred automatically overnight to the REDCap's common pool of patients' database. Further rules were developed to sort the patients automatically based on laboratory, pathological, surgical techniques, or possible diagnoses. This allowed access to patient's data on the research nurses' interface. These nurses now open medical records and verify the diagnoses. Once they choose that the diagnosis had been verified, the particular patient's data appear on the designated CRAs/CRSs view. The CRAs/CRSs start preparing clinical trial consents, complementing the case report forms, and preparing patient's educational materials. Patients who require special attention or a deviation from protocols are highlighted due to other applied rules. Both automatic and manual data collection and validation cycles continue by the end of treatment and over follow-up milestones. Upon data analysis time point, the data gathering is conducted based on designated filtering rules and exported in the forms of interpretable data formats by data analysis software that helps develop more customizable reports and publishing-ready graphs. Data are concomitantly shared with the national cancer registries. Daily exports of patient datasets and their confirmed diagnoses are shared

with the hospital biobank and epidemiology team to start preparing consents, filling custom forms, and collecting samples. The workflow of the publishing process has been accelerated dramatically after the mentioned implementations.

All in all, the founding of the cancer registry has provided a "safe haven" of complete and reliable patient's data for scientists and researchers. Elsewhere, the lack of solid patient's data continues to hinder quality medical research. The establishment of this registry has thus laid the groundwork for more complex and more ambitious studies to be carried out in the near future.

Acknowledgments I would like to thank Dr. Mohamed-Ismail Rakha and Dr. Uta Schmidt-Straßburger for revising the chapter and my friend Mohamed Sabry for giving ideas for it. Mohamed Sabry has led the cancer registry efforts mentioned in the chapter supervised by Dr. Sameera Ezzat. Moreover, I want to thank the Ruth und Adolf Merckle endowment fund for the financial support of my Oncology studies between 2012 and 2014 at the University of Ulm.

References

Alfaar AS, Hassan WM, Bakry MS, Qaddoumi I (2017a) Neonates with cancer and causes of death; lessons from 615 cases in the SEER databases. Cancer Med 6:1817–1826

Alfaar AS, Nour R, Bakry MS et al (2017b) A change roadmap towards research paradigm in low-resource countries: retinoblastoma model in Egypt. Int Ophthalmol 37:111–118

Alfaar AS, Saad A, Elzouki S et al (2020) Uveal melanoma-associated cancers revisited. ESMO Open 5:e000990. https://doi.org/10.1136/esmoopen-2020-000990

Amgad M, AlFaar AS (2014) Integrating web 2.0 in clinical research education in a developing country. J Cancer Educ 29:536–540. https://doi.org/10.1007/s13187-013-0595-5

Armstrong BK (1992) The role of the cancer registry in cancer control. Cancer Causes Control 3:569–579. https://doi.org/10.1007/BF00052754

Glicksberg BS, Burns S, Currie R et al (2020) Blockchain-authenticated sharing of genomic and clinical outcomes data of patients with cancer: a prospective cohort study. J Med Internet Res 22:e16810. https://doi.org/10.2196/16810

Harbour JW, Onken MD, Roberson EDO et al (2010) Frequent mutation of BAP1 in metastasizing uveal melanomas. Science 330:1410–1413. https://doi.org/10.1126/science.1194472

Harris PA, Taylor R, Thielke R et al (2009) Research electronic data capture (REDCap)—a metadata-driven methodology and workflow process for providing translational research informatics support. J Biomed Inform 42:377–381. https://doi.org/10.1016/j.jbi.2008.08.010

Hassan WM, Alfaar AS, Bakry MS, Ezzat S (2014) Orbital tumors in USA: difference in survival patterns. Cancer Epidemiol 38:515–522. https://doi.org/10.1016/j.canep.2014.07.001

Hassan WM, Bakry MS, Hassan HM, Alfaar AS (2016) Incidence of orbital, conjunctival and lacrimal gland malignant tumors in USA from surveillance, epidemiology and end results, 1973-2009. Int J Ophthalmol 9:1808–1813. https://doi.org/10.18240/ijo.2016.12.18

Hofferkamp J (2008) Standards for completeness, quality, analysis, management, security and confidentiality of data. In: Standards for cancer registries, vol Vol. 3. North American Association of Central Cancer Registries, Springfield, IL

Izquierdo JN, Schoenbach VJ (2000) The potential and limitations of data from population-based state cancer registries. Am J Public Health 90:695–698. https://doi.org/10.2105/ajph.90.5.695

Jensen OM, Parkin DM, MacLennan R et al (1991) Cancer registration: principles and methods (IARC Scientific Publications). Oxford University Press, New York

Kumar A, Guss ZD, Courtney PT et al (2020) Evaluation of the use of cancer registry data for comparative effectiveness research. JAMA Netw Open 3:e2011985. https://doi.org/10.1001/jamanetworkopen.2020.11985

Labib RM, Mostafa MM, Alfaar AS et al (2016) Biorepository for pediatric cancer with minimal resources: meeting the challenges. Biopreserv Biobank 14:9–16. https://doi.org/10.1089/bio.2015.0004

Menck H, Smart CR (1994) Central cancer registries: design, management, and use. Harwood-Academic Publishers, Chur

Parkin DM (2006) The evolution of the population-based cancer registry. Nat Rev Cancer 6:603–612. https://doi.org/10.1038/nrc1948

Saad AM, Gad MM, Al-Husseini MJ et al (2018) Suicidal death within a year of a cancer diagnosis: a population-based study. Cancer. https://doi.org/10.1002/cncr.31876

Terry NP (2012) Protecting patient privacy in the age of big data. UMKC L Rev 81:385

The International Agency for Research on Cancer (IARC) (n.d.) Global Cancer Observatory Resources. https://gco.iarc.fr/resources.php. Accessed 25 Apr 2021

Whippen D, Deering MJ, Ambinder EP (2007) Advancing high-quality cancer care: cancer biomedical informatics grid supports personalized medicine and the electronic health record. J Oncol Pract 3:208–211. https://doi.org/10.1200/JOP.0743501

Zekri W, Yehia D, Elshafie MM et al (2015) Bilateral clear cell sarcoma of the kidney. J Egypt Natl Canc Inst 27:97–100

Asking Existing Data the Right Questions: Data Mining as a Research Option in Low- and Middle-Income Countries

Velizar Shivarov

Background

I graduated as medical doctor from the Medical University in my home country (Bulgaria) in 2003. At that time, Bulgaria was on its way to join two important international unions (NATO and EU), which were expected to define its long-term political orientation and the rapid establishment of democratic values in all domains of the Bulgarian society. During my studies, I have developed a genuine interest in science and was eager to have an opportunity to pursue an academic career with some research focus. I was quite unsure how to find a pathway in experimental medicine as in Bulgaria the medical education is primarily focused on clinical practice. However, shortly afterward, I was able to win a scholarship by the Japanese government (MEXT scholarship) and was hosted by the leading immunologist Tasuku Honjo. I spent 18 months in Kyoto and realized the power of molecular medicine, and I was fascinated by the central dogma in molecular biology (Crick 1970), that is, that life itself is a flow of information between macromolecules, and it is our ability to understand and decode this information in order to achieve a comprehensive understanding of living matter. Upon my leave from Kyoto, I was firmly determined to follow Prof. Honjo's advice "always to follow my research questions and to try to stay close to science" (Fig. 1). I spent the next several years in Bulgaria and the USA developing skills and expertise in immunology and hematology. In 2012, I started the Master Online Advanced Oncology Study Program at Ulm University, which provided me with a broader conceptual view on cancer and triggered me to develop further skills in biostatistics and big data analysis. In that respect, I found really transforming the lessons by Prof. Dietrich Rothenbacher and my MSc thesis advisor Prof. Lars Bullinger.

At that time, I have already been based in Bulgaria and was struggling to perform some high-quality research. Indeed, there were two main problems that I faced. Bulgaria was and still is lagging behind most of the countries in the EU in terms of spending on R&D both in absolute numbers and as a percentage of GDP (http://uis.unesco.org/apps/visualisations/research-and-development-spending/). Furthermore, the only governmental organization responsible for research funding was suffering from a series of malpractices (https://www.nature.com/news/2011/110406/full/472019a.html). Because of those hurdles, I realized that one of the reasonable ways to perform good quality research is to make use of existing data sources. To follow that goal, I invested additional efforts in developing skills in big data analysis. That was achievable

V. Shivarov (✉)
Faculty of Biology, Department of Genetics, St. Kliment Ohridski Sofia University, Sofia, Bulgaria

PRAHS, Sofia, Bulgaria

U. Schmidt-Strassburger (ed.), *Improving Oncology Worldwide*, Sustainable Development Goals Series, https://doi.org/10.1007/978-3-030-96053-7_9

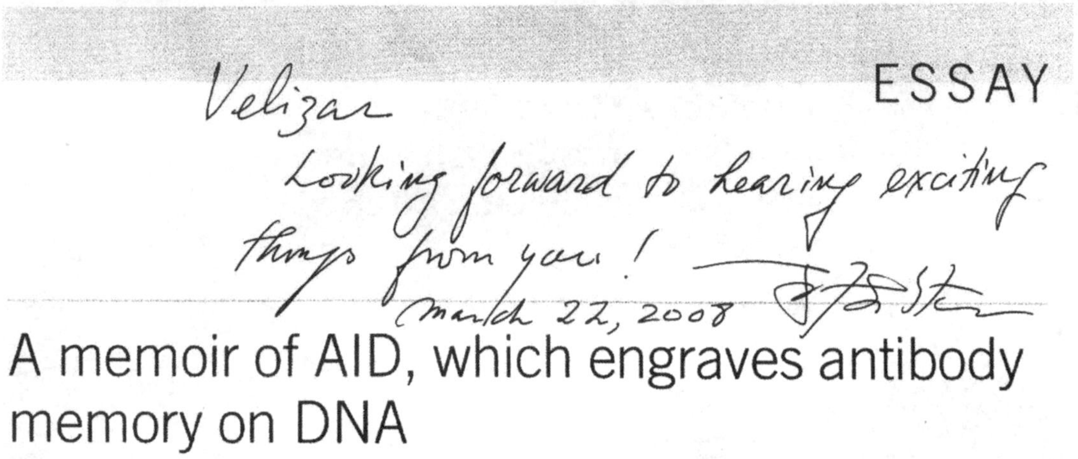

ESSAY

Velizar
Looking forward to hearing exciting
things from you !
March 22, 2008

A memoir of AID, which engraves antibody memory on DNA

Tasuku Honjo

Tasuku Honjo recounts his work aimed at unraveling the molecular mystery of how antibodies undergo antigen-induced maturation.

Fig. 1 A copy of a small gift from Prof. Tasuku Honjo, which made me obliged to try to pursue my own research questions

because of the accessibility of a series of MOOCs (massive open online courses) in biostatistics and big data analysis on Coursera (www.coursera.org) and edX (www.edx.org) platforms. Further to that, I developed my clinical skills in hematology and became a certified clinical hematologist as well as theoretical concepts in cancer biology through participation in another blended learning course (https://postgraduateeducation.hms.harvard.edu/certificate-programs/research-programs/high-impact-cancer-research). The latter helped me shape my understanding of cancer research in the context of cancer hallmarks (Hanahan and Weinberg 2011) and their application in malignant hematology and cancer immunology (Alkhazraji et al. 2019). With such a set of skills and conceptual background, I was able to address various topics in several directions as outlined below.

Prognostic Values of Different Mutations in Acute Myeloid Leukemia (AML)

While participating in the Master Online Advanced Oncology Study Program, there was a debate on the prognostic value of several newly identified mutations in AML patients. Several cooperative groups had started to publish their retrospective analyses. Inspired by the Biometrics module of the program, I decided to address the prognostic role of *DNMT3A* mutations in adult AML patients. I self-learned how to use the most popular software for that purpose (RevMan) and included 9 studies with over 4500 AML cases and almost 1000 *DNMT3A* mutated cases (Shivarov et al. 2013). Our meta-analysis showed that *DNMT3A* mutations conferred significantly worse prognosis with both shorter overall and relapse free survival (Shivarov et al. 2013). This prognostic value was independent of the cytogenetic features of AML. Our findings were later confirmed by other groups' meta-analyses (Tie et al. 2014; Ahn et al. 2016).

After that initial experience, I focused on the prognostic value of *ASXL1* mutations. Analogous to our experience with *DNMT3A* mutations, we performed meta-analysis on 6 studies with over 3300 patients (including 307 *ASXL1* mutated cases) (Shivarov et al. 2015). Notably, we demonstrated that *ASXL1* mutations conferred a worse prognosis in both younger and older patients (Shivarov et al. 2015). We extended the study by performing a meta-analysis of gene expression data in order to obtain a robust gene expression profile associated with the presence of *ASXL1* mutations. Gene ontology analysis showed that *ASXL1* mutations were associated with catabolic processes and phosphatase activity (Shivarov et al. 2015).

Outcomes Research Using Data from Cancer Registries

Population-based cancer registries can be invaluable sources of raw data for epidemiological and outcomes research. The largest registry providing free data access is the Surveillance, Epidemiology, and End Results (SEER) Program (www.seer. cancer.gov). Although the SEER database does not provide in-depth data on histological features, imaging, and therapy, it does provide data on date of diagnosis, demographic and social characteristics, secondary cancers, cause of death, and survival data allowing a number of possible analyses. Free access to the latest release of SEER database was then granted upon individual application without specifying the specific project the data will be used for. These days, a straightforward process provides access to this valuable source. The granted access comes along with the SEERStat software which allows for a number of predefined statistical analyses. Another approach is to perform a case listing through filtering based on various criteria and to perform a subsequent descriptive or inferential statistics with commercial or free software tools. In the last several years, we used the SEER to perform outcomes research in a number of rare hematological malignancies. We analyzed the clinical outcomes of nodular lymphocyte-predominant Hodgkin lymphoma (NLPHL) after the year 2000 (Shivarov and Ivanova 2018). We listed 1401 such cases and were able to demonstrate that there was no difference in survival between males and females, which was suggested by some previous reports (Shivarov and Ivanova 2018). Furthermore, the introduction of rituximab in the management of this disease in the mid-2000s appeared not to affect clinical prognosis (Shivarov and Ivanova 2018). In line with this

study, we also used cases listed from the SEER database to identify a significant number of cases with either composite or sequential B-cell lymphomas with features intermediate between DLBCL/PMBCL and classical Hodgkin lymphoma (Shivarov and Ivanova 2020). We demonstrated differences in overall survival between composite and sequential lymphomas (Shivarov and Ivanova 2020). We also showed that the order of the type of B-cell lymphomas in sequential lymphoma cases also has prognostic impact (Shivarov and Ivanova 2020). Collectively, the data from this study demonstrated how to use registry data to define new entities and to address in an unbiased fashion the role of some factors on clinical outcomes. Another small study that we performed addressed the incidence of secondary malignancies in classical HL after the year 2000 (presented at EHA Annual Congress in 2018). We also assessed the risk of second solid cancers in another rare hematologic malignancy—systemic mastocytosis (SM) (Shivarov et al. 2018). SM with an associated hematologic neoplasm is a well-defined SM subgroup, but at the time of our analysis, it was not reported whether SM was associated with an increased risk for solid cancers as well. Notably, based on the SEER data SM cases, we could not identify a consistently increased risk for second solid cancers (Shivarov et al. 2018).

Using Publicly Available Omics Datasets to Build or Support Original Hypotheses

I have had a genuine interest in the molecular biology of Philadelphia chromosome-negative myeloproliferative neoplasms (MPNs) since 2005 after the identification of JAK2 V617F mutation as the most frequent mutation in all three classical MPNs—essential thrombocythemia (ET), polycythemia vera (PV), and primary myelofibrosis (PMF) (Kralovics et al. 2005; Levine et al. 2005; Vainchenker and Constantinescu 2005; Baxter et al. 2005). Indeed, over the years, we developed several multiplex methods for the detection of mutations in myeloid malignancies including

JAK2 V617F (Shivarov et al. 2011). In December 2013, I had the opportunity to listen to the original reports of the identification of the second most frequent group of MPN-associated mutations—those in exon 9 of the calreticulin gene (CALR) (Klampfl et al. 2013; Nangalia et al. 2013). I was struck by the invariable common neoformed C-terminus that all those frameshift mutations caused. Two ideas were particularly appealing to me: (i) that the structural characteristics of the neoformed C-terminus may play a role in its mechanism of neoplastic transformation; and (ii) this unique C-terminus is probably a new source of variable neoepitopes. To address the former idea, we performed bioinformatic analyses of the sequence of the neoformed C-terminus and proposed that it was structurally disordered and cannot bind Ca^{2+}, which would have direct mechanistic and therapeutic implications (Shivarov et al. 2014). The second idea was further developed so that we reached to a project assessing the role of immunoediting in MPNs. We initially questioned whether protective HLA alleles for the development of JAK2 V617F+ MPNs existed. We genotyped a large number of MPN patients and healthy controls and demonstrated that two HLA class I alleles were significantly less frequent in JAK2 V617F+ patients in comparison to healthy individuals. Interestingly, we used a bioinformatic approach to show that the HLA-B*35:01 allele can bind a specific 9-mer peptide derived from the mutant JAK2 protein (NetMHCpan server) (Ivanova et al. 2020). Using other bioinformatic tools, we were also able to show that the same peptide was likely to be successfully processed and presented in the HLA class I antigen processing and presentation pathway. Therefore, we proposed that adaptive immune response through cognate T cells can edit early carcinogenesis in JAK2 V617F+ MPN stem cells (MPN-SCs) in the presence of alleles such as HLA-B*35:01, which are able to present JAK2 V617F-derived peptides efficiently (Fig. 2) (Ivanova et al. 2020). The major criticism of that hypothesis would be that the protection is not absolute and JAK2 V617F+ MPNs can still develop even in the presence of potentially protective HLA class I alleles. We therefore proposed

that MPN-SCs can escape immunoediting through downregulation of important genes in the HLA class I antigen processing and presentation pathway (Fig. 2). We did not have our own expression data, so we sought to provide such evidence using publicly available datasets. We were able to show that bone marrow (BM)-derived CD34+ cells from PV and ET downregulated key components of antigen processing and presentation machinery, including HLA-A and HLA-B (Ivanova et al. 2020). The same phenomenon was not observed in PMF and PV peripheral blood (PB) CD34+ cells. We further analyzed the effect of various treatments on HLA gene expression. Notably, short-term ruxolitinib treatment JAK2 V617F+ CD34+ SET-2 cell line was associated with an upregulation of some HLA genes such as HLA-A, HLA-E, and HLA-F (Ivanova et al. 2020). On the other hand, SET-2 cells that persisted long-term ruxolitinib treatment showed a downregulation of HLA-A, HLA-B, HLA-C, HLA-E, and HLA-G. Analogous to ruxolitinib, we showed that short-term treatment of JAK2 V617F+ mouse cells with IFN-α led to upregulation of most genes of the MHC-I pathway (Ivanova et al. 2020). However, long-term treatment with IFN-α in vivo did not show changes in the expression of MHC class I pathway genes in mouse long-term HSCs (Ivanova et al. 2020).

Collectively, our own genetic data, bioinformatic predictions, and analysis of a number of publicly available gene expression datasets allowed us to propose a model of immunoediting in the early pathogenesis of JAK2 V617F+ MPNs (Fig. 2) (Ivanova et al. 2020).

Conclusions

Several personal milestones in the last 15 years helped me shape my understanding of scientific medicine. My participation in the Advanced Oncology Program at Ulm University was one of them and just confirmed the lesson I got earlier from my first scientific mentor Prof. Tasuku Honjo that in order to succeed in science, you "must work hard, be smart, and have a devoted mentor." The difficulties in my career afterward

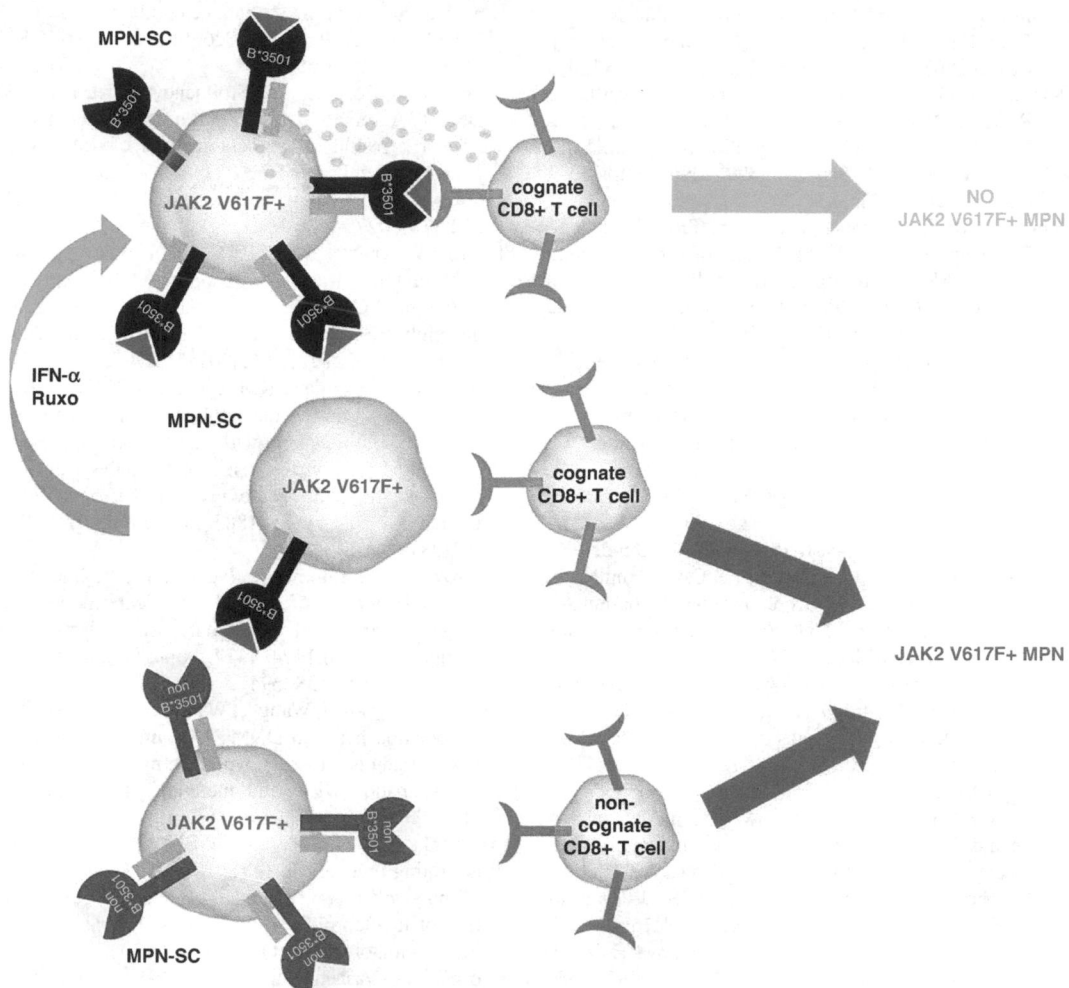

Fig. 2 Our proposed model for the HLA-mediated immunoediting in JAK2 V516F+ MPNs. Modified from Ivanova et al. (Ivanova et al. 2020)

made me realize that the program was an important preparation to face those challenges, as after all "the fact that you dare swim against the mainstream means that you have already become a very good swimmer."

References

Ahn J-S, Kim H-J, Kim Y-K, Lee S-S, Jung S-H, Yang D-H et al (2016) DNMT3A R882 mutation with FLT3-ITD positivity is an extremely poor prognostic factor in patients with normal-karyotype acute myeloid leukemia after allogeneic hematopoietic cell transplantation. Biol Blood Marrow Transplant 22(1):61–70

Alkhazraji A, Elgamal M, Ang SH, Shivarov V (2019) All cancer hallmarks lead to diversity. Int J Clin Exp Med 12(1):132–157

Baxter EJ, Scott LM, Campbell PJ, East C, Fourouclas N, Swanton S et al (2005) Acquired mutation of the tyrosine kinase JAK2 in human myeloproliferative disorders. Lancet 365(9464):1054–1061. https://doi.org/10.1016/S0140-6736(05)71142-9. S0140-6736(05)71142-9 [pii]

Crick F (1970) Central dogma of molecular biology. Nature 227(5258):561–563. https://doi.org/10.1038/227561a0

Hanahan D, Weinberg RA (2011) Hallmarks of cancer: the next generation. Cell 144(5):646–674. https://doi.org/10.1016/j.cell.2011.02.013. S0092-8674(11)00127-9 [pii]

Ivanova M, Tsvetkova G, Lukanov T, Stoimenov A, Hadjiev E, Shivarov V (2020) Probable HLA-mediated immunoediting of JAK2 V617F-driven oncogenesis. Exp Hematol 92:75–88. https://doi.org/10.1016/j.exphem.2020.09.200. S0301-472X(20)30565-8 [pii]

Klampfl T, Gisslinger H, Harutyunyan AS, Nivarthi H, Rumi E, Milosevic JD et al (2013) Somatic mutations of calreticulin in myeloproliferative neoplasms. N Engl J Med 369(25):2379–2390. https://doi.org/10.1056/NEJMoa1311347

Kralovics R, Passamonti F, Buser AS, Teo SS, Tiedt R, Passweg JR et al (2005) A gain-of-function mutation of JAK2 in myeloproliferative disorders. N Engl J Med 352(17):1779–1790. https://doi.org/10.1056/NEJMoa051113. 352/17/1779 [pii]

Levine RL, Wadleigh M, Cools J, Ebert BL, Wernig G, Huntly BJ et al (2005) Activating mutation in the tyrosine kinase JAK2 in polycythemia vera, essential thrombocythemia, and myeloid metaplasia with myelofibrosis. Cancer Cell 7(4):387–397. https://doi.org/10.1016/j.ccr.2005.03.023. S1535-6108(05)00094-2 [pii]

Nangalia J, Massie CE, Baxter EJ, Nice FL, Gundem G, Wedge DC et al (2013) Somatic CALR mutations in myeloproliferative neoplasms with nonmutated JAK2. N Engl J Med 369(25):2391–2405. https://doi.org/10.1056/NEJMoa1312542

Shivarov V, Ivanova M (2018) Nodular lymphocyte predominant Hodgkin lymphoma in USA between 2000 and 2014: an updated analysis based on the SEER data. Br J Haematol 182(5):727–730. https://doi.org/10.1111/bjh.14861

Shivarov V, Ivanova M (2020) Clinical outcomes of composite and sequential B-cell lymphomas with features intermediate between DLBCL/PMBCL and classical Hodgkin lymphoma from the SEER database. Br J Haematol 190(3):464–466. https://doi.org/10.1111/bjh.16728

Shivarov V, Ivanova M, Hadjiev E, Naumova E (2011) Rapid quantification of JAK2 V617F allele burden using a bead-based liquid assay with locked nucleic acid-modified oligonucleotide probes. Leuk Lymphoma 52(10):2023–2026. https://doi.org/10.3109/10428194.2011.584995

Shivarov V, Gueorguieva R, Stoimenov A, Tiu R (2013) DNMT3A mutation is a poor prognosis biomarker in AML: results of a meta-analysis of 4500 AML patients. Leuk Res 37(11):1445–1450. https://doi.org/10.1016/j.leukres.2013.07.032. S0145-2126(13)00275-0 [pii]

Shivarov V, Ivanova M, Tiu RV (2014) Mutated calreticulin retains structurally disordered C terminus that cannot bind Ca(2+): some mechanistic and therapeutic implications. Blood Cancer J 4:e185. https://doi.org/10.1038/bcj.2014.7. bcj20147 [pii]

Shivarov V, Gueorguieva R, Ivanova M, Tiu RV (2015) ASXL1 mutations define a subgroup of patients with acute myeloid leukemia with distinct gene expression profile and poor prognosis: a meta-analysis of 3311 adult patients with acute myeloid leukemia. Leuk Lymphoma 56(6):1881–1883. https://doi.org/10.3109/10428194.2014.974596

Shivarov V, Gueorguieva R, Ivanova M, Stoimenov A (2018) Incidence of second solid cancers in mastocytosis patients: a SEER database analysis. Leuk Lymphoma 59(6):1474–1477. https://doi.org/10.1080/10428194.2017.1382694

Tie R, Zhang T, Fu H, Wang L, Wang Y, He Y et al (2014) Association between DNMT3A mutations and prognosis of adults with de novo acute myeloid leukemia: a systematic review and meta-analysis. PLoS One 9(6):e93353

Vainchenker W, Constantinescu SN (2005) A unique activating mutation in JAK2 (V617F) is at the origin of polycythemia vera and allows a new classification of myeloproliferative diseases. Hematology Am Soc Hematol Educ Program 195-200. https://doi.org/10.1182/asheducation-2005.1.195. 2005/1/195 [pii]

Molecular and Cellular Analyses of Breast Cancers in Real Life

Carlos A. Castaneda

Introduction

Breast cancer is the most common women's malignancy in the world and in South American countries, including Peru, and it is the leading cause of cancer-related death in women. Different reports indicate that race and a country's income can influence prognosis in breast cancer. Part of these disparities is because women from low-income countries have a delay in cancer management and are diagnosed with more advanced stages. However, different publications also describe that rates of aggressive tumor features have a higher prevalence in some races (Castaneda et al. 2018).

Biomarkers in Breast Cancer

As we are entering the era of personalized medicine, much attention has been paid to identify biomarkers of prognosis and response to therapies targeting a tumor's genetic background (André et al. 2019).

One of the most immediate challenges after diagnosis is to identify who should receive adjuvant treatment and to select the most suitable therapy in early stages and how to choose the most effective and least toxic therapy in advanced disease. A substantial amount of research has been invested in the development and validation of prognostic factors and predictive biomarkers.

A good biomarker should be analytically valid, reproducible, and respond to a relevant clinical question. It must also be affordable and accessible to pathologists and laboratory scientists in both academic and community practice centers worldwide to be incorporated into daily practice (Fig. 1) (Salgado et al. 2019).

Biomarkers in Cancer Cells

The most recognized prognostic tumor factors in early breast cancer are the two macroscopic pathological features, regional lymph node metastases and tumor size, and the microscopic feature tumor grade. Histology grade is widely informed based on the Nottingham system. This system utilizes three microscopic features: nuclear pleomorphism, gland or tubule formation, and the number of dividing cells.

Detection of estrogen receptor (ER), progesterone receptor (PgR), HER2, and the widely used Ki67 index has become a requirement for choosing the treatment through the worldwide cancer centers (Rebaza et al. 2018). Although the last one has been described as having a poor interlaboratory precision and lack of a validated cutoff point, the International Ki67 in the Breast

C. A. Castaneda (✉)
Department of Medical Oncology, Instituto Nacional de Enfermedades Neoplásicas, Lima, Peru

© The Author(s) 2022
U. Schmidt-Strassburger (ed.), *Improving Oncology Worldwide*, Sustainable Development Goals Series,
https://doi.org/10.1007/978-3-030-96053-7_10

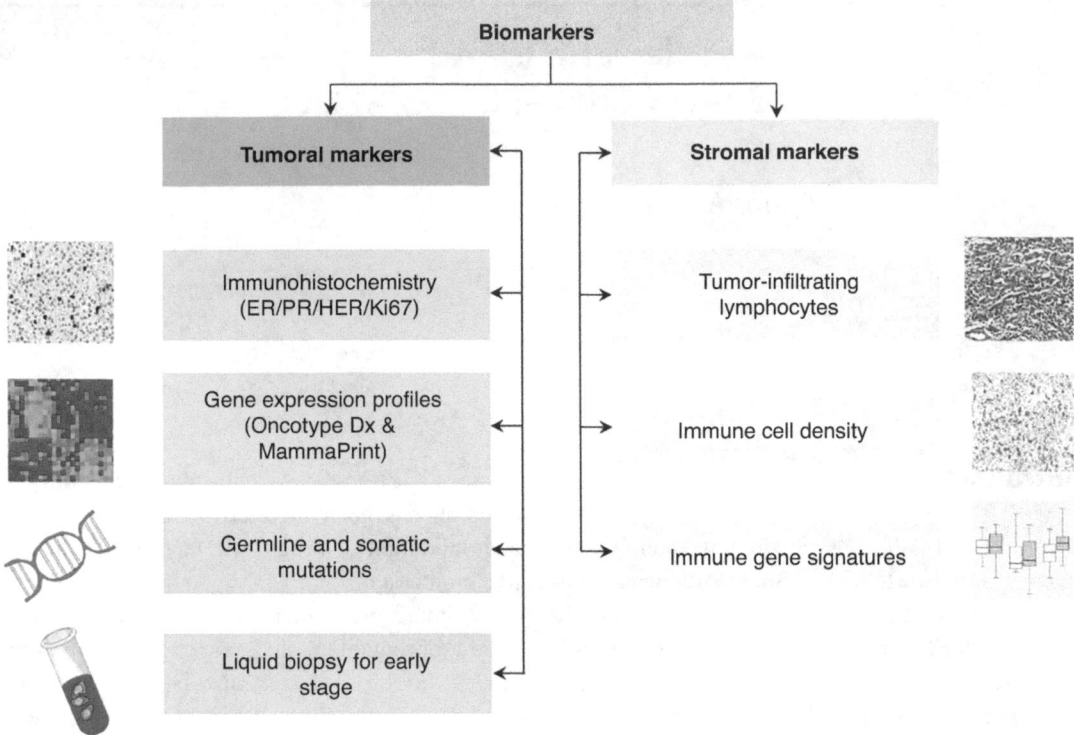

Fig. 1 Biomarkers in breast cancer

Cancer Working Group makes technical recommendations for improving assay results and indicates that <5% and >30% Ki67 counts have better interlaboratory precision (Nielsen et al. 2021).

The American Society of Clinical Oncology (ASCO)/College of American Pathologists (CAP) periodically reviews the guidelines for cataloging ER and PgR, and the last actualization was performed in 2020. They categorize positive status for ER or PgR when 1–100% of tumor nuclei positive are found. The low ER-positive status is demonstrated when 1%–10% of tumor cell nuclei are immunoreactive (Allison et al. 2020).

Similarly, a periodical review of the guidelines for HER2 status is performed and the last was done in 2018. It classifies the status as positive when the IHC result is 3+ and negative if the IHC result is 0 or 1+. If the IHC result is 2+ (weak to moderate complete membrane staining observed in <10% of tumor cells), a dual ISH or FISH is recommended to be performed. Combination between HER2/CEP17 ratio and

mean HER2 copy number can fit in one of five scenarios. The first (HER2/CEP17 ratio ≥ 2.0 and average HER2 copy number ≥ 4.0) and the third scenarios (HER2/CEP17 ratio < 2.0 and HER2 copy number of ≥ 6) are classified as positive (Wolff et al. 2018).

There have been described other immunohistochemistry biomarkers like androgen receptor, and their analysis has been described by my group at the Peruvian Cancer Institute in a local series of 95 triple-negative breast cancer (TNBC) samples (Castaneda et al. 2019).

Additionally, platforms of tumor gene expression have demonstrated their prognostic value and some of them a predictive role for adjuvant treatment (Sparano et al. 2018; Cardoso et al. 2020; Müller et al. 2021; Gnant et al. 2015). Oncotype Dx is the most widely used multigene signature for predicting outcome in breast cancer, and the tool is available in the different continents. It tests 21 genes at the mRNA level by using RT-PCR, including 16 linked to cancer, and provides quantification of gene expression for

ER, PgR, and HER2. It generates a recurrence score (RS) as a continuous variable that divides patients into prognostic groups as well as benefit from adjuvant chemotherapy. The prospective trial TAILORx with more than 10,000 node-negative breast cancer cases demonstrated that there was a low risk of recurrence after endocrine therapy alone in patients with RS = 0–10. The endocrine therapy alone was noninferior to adjuvant chemotherapy plus endocrine therapy in the overall population with RS = 11–25 and a high likelihood of benefit from chemotherapy in patients with RS = 26–100. A chemotherapy benefit was noted in patients ≤50 years old with an RS of 16–25 (Sparano et al. 2018). A new tool (RSClin) that integrates RS with tumor grade, tumor size, and age has demonstrated its value to predict chemotherapy benefit (Sparano et al. 2021). Recent analyses find that race influences the value of the test, and Black women had worse clinical outcomes despite similar RS (Hoskins et al. 2021). Finally, the recently presented RxPONDER trial enrolled 5015 stage II/stage III breast cancer patients and found that postmenopausal women with ER-positive, HER2-negative breast cancer with 1–3 positive nodes and RS ≤ 25 derived no benefit from adding chemotherapy to endocrine therapy. On the other side, premenopausal women experience a 46% reduction in recurrence risk with the addition of chemotherapy (Müller et al. 2021).

MammaPrint assay is another platform that is a microarray-based technique that evaluates a 70-gene signature related to proliferation, invasion, and angiogenesis. The MINDACT trial is a phase III trial evaluating 6693 node-negative and 1–3 node-positive early breast cancer patients that demonstrated to have better prognostic value than the evaluation using standard clinicopathological features. A recent long-term analysis confirmed the prognostic value of the tool in women >50 years (Cardoso et al. 2020).

Determination of germline mutations including BRCA1, BRCA2, and other genes related to DNA repair mechanisms has been largely associated with hereditary breast cancer, and somatic mutations in similar genes have similarly been described in tumor lesions. Their presence has been described as predictive for response to platinum chemotherapy and enzyme-poly-ADP-ribose-polymerase inhibitor compounds. The methodology for their detection has also been recently implemented in South American countries, and the experience in their interpretation is increasingly required in daily practice (Castaneda et al. 2018; Oliver et al. 2019; Oh et al. 2021).

Circulating Biomarkers

The analysis of compounds in blood such as CA15-3 and CEA has all been shown to predict poor outcome in patients with breast cancer (Molina et al. 2010).

Several studies have shown that somatic mutations identified in ctDNA are widely representative of the tumor genome and can provide an alternative noninvasive method that overcomes many difficulties related to tissue biopsy. The detection of mutation in the ligand-binding domain of ESR1 in ctDNA that confers constitutive activity of ER is an emerging predictor of endocrine therapy resistance in the metastatic setting. ctDNA levels also closely reflect changes in tumor burden and can predict the progressive disease several months before the standard imaging. Levels of ctDNA may also be an important indicator of prognosis; however, prospective studies in larger cohorts of patients are still needed to validate their prognostic role. CTCs are cancer cells that have been shed or actively migrate into the vasculature from the primary tumor or metastatic lesions and circulate in the bloodstream. They can give rise to metastases (seeding hypothesis) in distant organs (Stanton et al. 2016; Denkert et al. 2018). CTC enumeration has demonstrated to have a prognostic value in the metastatic setting and to predict early and late recurrences as well as shorter overall survival (OS) in early breast cancer. Beyond enumeration, there is interest in genotypic and phenotypic characterization of CTCs that may help in revealing the underlying mechanism of tumorigenesis and metastases. In contrast to CTCs, a cutoff of ctDNA that correlates with a worse prognosis has not been identified yet (Rossi et al. 2018).

During the last 4 years, we have been working in the detection of ctDNA through digital PCR equipment in plasma samples from 183 breast cancer patients. We found a PIK3CA mutation in ctDNA in 35% cases (most with E545K), and it was associated with lower levels of tumor-infiltrating lymphocytes (TILs) ($p = 0.04$). PIK3CA in ctDNA tended to be associated with advanced stages ($p = 0.09$) in whole series and with higher recurrence rates ($p = 0.053$) in the nonmetastatic setting. Patients with presence of PIK3CA mutations in their ctDNA tend to have shorter OS ($p = 0.083$) (Galvez-Nino et al. 2020).

Biomarkers in Stromal Cells

Malignant cell transformation alters the structure of cell membrane proteins and induces antitumor responses against tumor antigens which eliminate the developing tumor cells. Dendritic cells can take antigens and migrate to lymphoid organs, where they present their antigens to adaptive immune cells.

Effector T-cells include various subsets: T helper cells, T helper 1 (TH1), TH2 cells, TH17 cells, regulatory T (Treg) cells, T follicular helper cells, and cytotoxic T lymphocytes (CTLs).

TH1 cells produce cytokines, such as IFN-gamma and IL-2, which play important roles in activating and regulating the CTL responses. Meanwhile, TH2 cells secrete cytokines that stimulate humoral immune responses as well as IL-4 and IL-10 which downregulate the pro-inflammatory state and inhibit the synthesis of TH1 cytokines.

CTLs confer cytolytic activity by releasing perforin and other cytotoxins that induce apoptosis. The antitumor activation of T-cells relies on T-cell receptor (TCR) recognition of antigenic peptides presented by major histocompatibility complex molecules on the neoplastic cells.

However, tumors have developed some mechanisms inhibiting T-cell responses. Upregulation of CTLA-4 in CD8+ T-cells produces an inhibitory effect over the stimulatory activity of the CD28 receptor after TCR engagement with antigens. Another inhibitory receptor in T-cells is

PD-1 that is activated by their ligand PD-L1 which can be upregulated by tumor cells. In addition, there are inhibitory cells present in the tumor microenvironment, including M2-polarized tumor-associated macrophages (TAMs) and Tregs. Tregs are identified as a population of CD4+ FOXP3+ T-cells that express CD25, a subunit of the receptor for the T-cell-stimulating cytokine IL-2, and also constitutively express CTLA-4. TAMs represent a highly heterogeneous immune cell population that express CD68 marker and have two polarized phenotypes, M1 and M2. The former is traditionally associated with antitumor effects and expresses CD80 and CD86, and the latter is typically showing protumorigenic characteristics and expresses CD163, CD204, and CD206.

Stromal tumor-infiltrating lymphocyte (TIL) level has been extensively described to be higher in triple-negative breast cancer (TNBC) and HER2+ than luminal phenotype (Stanton et al. 2016; Denkert et al. 2018). In addition, TIL levels are lower in metastatic and in heavily treated diseases, while levels are lower in tumor lesions located in the liver (Luen et al. 2017).

TILs have been strongly associated with prognosis in early-stage TNBC and HER2-positive breast cancer. Additionally, Denkert and colleagues found that TILs were independent predictors for pCR in an initial cohort ($n = 218$) and the validation set ($n = 840$). TIL-positive tumors achieved 40% and 42% of pCR, whereas the TIL-negative tumors achieved only 3%–7% pCR in the discovery and the validation cohort, respectively (Denkert et al. 2010).

A recent meta-analysis found that higher TIL levels predict pCR (OR 2.14, 95% CI 1.43–3.19) and longer OS (HR 0.9, CI 0.97–0.93) and DFS (disease-specific survival) (HR 0.66, 0.57–0.76) in the TNBC subset (Denkert et al. 2018; Gao et al. 2020; Loi et al. 2019).

Finally, an international collaboration network where we participated evaluated the role of TIL in residual lesions of TNBC. In a final series of 375 residual TNBC samples, TIL levels were significantly lower with increasing post-NAC tumor size, nodal stage but did not differ by residual cancer burden (RCB) class. Higher TIL in residual disease was associated with improved RFS ($p < 0.001$) and OS ($p < 0.001$). Greater magnitude of positive effect was observed for RCB class II than class III (Luen et al. 2019).

Therefore, TILs reached level 1b evidence as prognostic marker in early TNBC in the 16th St Gallen International Breast Cancer Consensus Conference. WHO (World Health Organization) and ESMO (European Society for Medical Oncology) also recommended their incorporation in the routine pathology report of early TNBC samples. However, TIL was not recommended for guiding systemic treatment selection (Burstein et al. 2019).

A large series of studies evaluated the prognostic significance of CD8+ T-cells in over 1300 breast cancer patients who underwent mastectomy or lumpectomy with radiation. The number of CD8+ T-cells correlated with a higher grade and inversely correlated with ER expression. In a multivariate model that included tumor size, stage, grade, vascular invasion, HER2 and ER status, age, and adjuvant treatment, the number of CD8+ T-cells was independently associated with improved disease-specific survival (DFS) ($p = 0.001$). This association keeps among the ER tumors but not in ER+ tumors (Mahmoud et al. 2011). A further geographic analysis of CD8 cell distribution inside the tumor lesions describes that fully infiltrated and stroma-restricted CD8+ infiltration had the most favorable prognosis (Gruosso et al. 2019). Other series of studies describe that CD8 expression can also have a negative effect over survival as is strongly correlated with FOXP3 expression (Bottai et al. 2016).

Garcia-Martinez et al. evaluated the role of CD3, CD4, CD8, CD20, CD68, and FOXP3 immune cells in pre- and post-neoadjuvant tumor samples in a series of 121 breast cancer patients in predicting response to neoadjuvant chemotherapy and survival. They found that higher pre-NAC infiltration by CD3, CD4, and CD20 was associated with pCR, and the predictive response role of CD4 was confirmed in six public genomic datasets. Higher CD68 density in residual post-NAC samples was associated with shorter OS. Analysis of the immune infiltrate in post-chemotherapy residual tumors identified a highly

CD3 and CD8 infiltrated profile with a worse DFS (García-Martínez et al. 2014).

A recent meta-analysis found that the CD4 TIL subgroup (high vs. low) showed a better OS (HR 0.49, 95% CI 0.32–0.76) and DFS (HR 0.54, 95% CI 0.36–0.8), and the CD8 TIL subgroup showed a better DFS (HR 0.55, 95% CI 0.38–0.81). FOXP3 TIL subgroup was associated with better DFS (HR 0.5, 95% CI 0.33–0.75) (Gao et al. 2020).

The predictive value of TIL over response to targeted therapy has been demonstrated for HER2 therapy and anti-PD1 checkpoint inhibitors. Loi and colleagues have evaluated the predictive value of TIL in 935 patients randomized between chemotherapies along with or without trastuzumab. They found that trastuzumab was not associated with decreased risk of relapse in patients without lymphocyte infiltration (HR, 1.0; 95% CI, 0.55–1.75; $p = 0.99$). The three-year DFS rate was 96% in patients with high TIL tumors treated with chemotherapy and trastuzumab (Loi et al. 2012).

Higher TIL levels were also found to predict longer DFS and reduction in recurrence rates in the ShortHER trial that compared 1 year or 9 weeks of trastuzumab duration in 866 cases. They also found that cases with TIL < 20% obtained significant benefit from the longer but not from shorter trastuzumab schedule (Dieci et al. 2019).

TILs were associated with DFS in the whole population from APHINITY phase III trial who received adjuvant pertuzumab or placebo added to standard chemotherapy/trastuzumab after resection in early HER2+ breast cancer (Krop et al. 2019).

Furthermore, TILs also correlate with outcome after immune checkpoint blockade in metastatic TNBC (Loi et al. 2017; Emens et al. 2019; Voorwerk et al. 2019).

The IMpassion130 trial evaluated the addition of atezolizumab to first-line chemotherapy with nab-paclitaxel in 902 metastatic TNBC patients, showing a significant PFS benefit in both the ITT population and the cohort with the presence of at least 1% staining of PD-L1 on immune cells. In addition, although OS was not significantly improved in the ITT, an increase in OS was observed among the PD-L1+ subgroups in the immunotherapy-containing arm (Schmid et al. 2018). Intratumoral CD8 were well correlated with PD-L1 and predicted progression-free survival (PFS) and OS; TILs had poor correlation with PD-L1 and were also associated with PFS but not OS (Emens et al. 2018). The KEYNOTE-355 trial evaluated the addition of pembrolizumab to three standard chemotherapeutic schedules in the first-line treatment of advanced TNBC. A significant PFS benefit was found with the addition of immunotherapy to first-line chemotherapy in the PD-L1+ population, defined by a combined positive score $\geq 10\%$ (Cortes et al. 2020).

There are two phase III randomized clinical trials that addressed the role of immune checkpoint inhibitors in the neoadjuvant setting of locally advanced TNBC. KEYNOTE-522 and IMpassion031 evaluated adding pembrolizumab or atezolizumab to standard neoadjuvant chemotherapy including anthracyclines. Although they demonstrated that the addition of antiPD1 therapy increased rates of pathologic complete response, they did not find that TIL levels or PD-L1 status predict the response (Schmid et al. 2020a,b; Loibl et al. 2019; Mittendorf et al. 2017, 2020).

After reviewing published information and analyzing our lab strengths and experience at the institute, a research team at the institute under collaboration with international research partners focused on evaluating the role of TIL levels and immune cell density in breast tumor samples before and after chemotherapy. After regulatory research issues, we evaluated 98 TNBC cases and found that higher TIL in pre-NST was associated with pathologic complete response and outcome. Post-NAC area with pCR had similar TIL levels than those without pCR ($p = 0.6331$). NAC produced a TIL decrease in full-face sections ($p < 0.0001$). Higher counts of CD3, CD4, CD8, and FOXP3 in pre-NAC samples had longer DFS. Higher counts of CD3 in pre-NAC samples had longer OS. Higher ratio of CD8/CD4 counts in pre-NAC was associated with pCR. Higher ratio of CD4/FOXP3 counts in pre-NAC was associated with longer DFS. Higher counts of CD4 in post-NAC area were associated with pCR (Castaneda et al. 2016).

Thereafter, we evaluated the role of TILs in 435 pre-NAC samples and found that they are associated with grade III, no luminal A subtype, RE negative, HER2 positive, and pCR (Galvez et al. 2018).

Conclusions

We can conclude that breast cancer is one of the most frequent malignancies, and biomarkers are allowing to improve treatment results. Technologies and procedures for evaluating biomarkers related to tumor cell behavior and their interaction with the stroma have been incorporated in the daily routine.

References

Allison KH, Hammond MEH, Dowsett M, McKernin SE, Carey LA, Fitzgibbons PL, et al. (2020) Estrogen and progesterone receptor testing in breast cancer: ASCO/CAP guideline update.

André F, Ciruelos E, Rubovszky G, Campone M, Loibl S, Rugo HS et al (2019) Alpelisib for PIK3CA-mutated, hormone receptor–positive advanced breast cancer. N Engl J Med 380(20):1929–1940

Bottai G, Raschioni C, Losurdo A, Di Tommaso L, Tinterri C, Torrisi R et al (2016) An immune stratification reveals a subset of PD-1/LAG-3 double-positive triple-negative breast cancers. Breast Cancer Res 18(1):1–10

Burstein HJ, Curigliano G, Loibl S, Dubsky P, Gnant M, Poortmans P et al (2019) Estimating the benefits of therapy for early-stage breast cancer: the St. Gallen international consensus guidelines for the primary therapy of early breast cancer 2019. Ann Oncol 30(10):1541–1557

Cardoso F, van't Veer L, Poncet C, Lopes Cardozo J, Delaloge S, Pierga J-Y et al (2020) MINDACT: long-term results of the large prospective trial testing the 70-gene signature MammaPrint as guidance for adjuvant chemotherapy in breast cancer patients. Am Soc Clin Oncol

Castaneda CA, Mittendorf E, Casavilca S, Wu Y, Castillo M, Arboleda P et al (2016) Tumor infiltrating lymphocytes in triple negative breast cancer receiving neoadjuvant chemotherapy. World J Clin Oncol 7(5)

Castaneda CA, Castillo M, Villarreal-Garza C, Rabanal C, Dunstan J, Calderon G et al (2018) Genetics, tumor features and treatment response of breast cancer in Latinas. Breast Cancer Manag 7(1):BMT01

Castaneda CA, Castillo M, Enciso JA, Enciso N, Bernabe LA, Sanchez J et al (2019) Role of undifferentiation markers and androgen receptor expression in triple-negative breast cancer. Breast J 25(6):1316

Cortes J, Cescon DW, Rugo HS, Nowecki Z, Im S-A, Yusof MM et al (2020) KEYNOTE-355: randomized, double-blind, phase III study of pembrolizumab+ chemotherapy versus placebo+ chemotherapy for previously untreated locally recurrent inoperable or metastatic triple-negative breast cancer. Am Soc Clin Oncol

Denkert C, Loibl S, Noske A, Roller M, Müller BM, Komor M et al (2010) Tumor-associated lymphocytes as an independent predictor of response to neoadjuvant chemotherapy in breast cancer. J Clin Oncol 28(1):105–113

Denkert C, von Minckwitz G, Darb-Esfahani S, Lederer B, Heppner BI, Weber KE et al (2018) Tumour-infiltrating lymphocytes and prognosis in different subtypes of breast cancer: a pooled analysis of 3771 patients treated with neoadjuvant therapy. Lancet Oncol 19(1):40–50

Dieci MV, Conte P, Bisagni G, Brandes AA, Frassoldati A, Cavanna L et al (2019) Association of tumor-infiltrating lymphocytes with distant disease-free survival in the ShortHER randomized adjuvant trial for patients with early HER2+ breast cancer. Ann Oncol 30(3):418–423

Emens LA, Loi S, Rugo HS, Schneeweiss A, Diéras V, Iwata H, et al. (2018) IMpassion130: efficacy in immune biomarker subgroups from the global, randomized, double-blind, placebo-controlled, phase III study of atezolizumab+ nab-paclitaxel in patients with treatment-naïve, locally advanced or metastatic triple-negative breast cancer. In: San Antonio Breast Cancer Symposium

Emens LA, Cruz C, Eder JP, Braiteh F, Chung C, Tolaney SM et al (2019) Long-term clinical outcomes and biomarker analyses of atezolizumab therapy for patients with metastatic triple-negative breast cancer: a phase 1 study. JAMA Oncol 5(1):74–82

Galvez M, Castaneda CA, Sanchez J, Castillo M, Rebaza LP, Calderon G et al (2018) Clinicopathological predictors of long-term benefit in breast cancer treated with neoadjuvant chemotherapy. World J Clin Oncol 9(2)

Galvez-Nino M, Roque K, Bernabe L, Garcia MC, Sanchez J, Valencia GGC et al (2020) 1991P detection of PIK3CA mutations in plasma samples at Peruvian cancer institute. Ann Oncol 31:S1114

Gao G, Wang Z, Qu X, Zhang Z (2020) Prognostic value of tumor-infiltrating lymphocytes in patients with triple-negative breast cancer: a systematic review and meta-analysis. BMC Cancer 20(1):1–15

García-Martínez E, Gil GL, Benito AC, González-Billalabeitia E, Conesa MAV, García TG et al (2014) Tumor-infiltrating immune cell profiles and their change after neoadjuvant chemotherapy predict response and prognosis of breast cancer. Breast Cancer Res 16(6):1–17

Gnant M, Sestak I, Filipits M, Dowsett M, Balic M, Lopez-Knowles E et al (2015) Identifying clinically relevant prognostic subgroups of postmenopausal women with node-positive hormone receptor-positive early-stage breast cancer treated with endocrine ther-

apy: a combined analysis of ABCSG-8 and ATAC using the PAM50 risk of recurrence. Ann Oncol 26(8):1685–1691

Gruosso T, Gigoux M, Manem VSK, Bertos N, Zuo D, Perlitch I et al (2019) Spatially distinct tumor immune microenvironments stratify triple-negative breast cancers. J Clin Invest 129(4):1785–1800

Hoskins KF, Danciu OC, Ko NY, Calip GS (2021) Association of Race/Ethnicity and the 21-Gene Recurrence Score With Breast Cancer–Specific Mortality Among US Women. JAMA Oncologia 7(3):370–378

Krop IE, Paulson J, Campbell C, Kiermaier AC, Andre F, Fumagalli D et al (2019) Genomic correlates of response to adjuvant trastuzumab (H) and pertuzumab (P) in HER2+ breast cancer (BC): biomarker analysis of the APHINITY trial. J Clin Oncol 37(15_suppl):1012–1012

Loi S, Michiels S, Lambrechts D, Salgado R, Sirtaine N, Fumagalli D et al (2012) Tumor PIK3CA mutations, lymphocyte infiltrrecurrence-free survival (RFS) in early breast cancer (BC): ation, and results from the FinHER trial. Am Soc Clin Oncol

Loi S, Adams S, Schmid P, Cortés J, Cescon DW, Winer EP et al (2017) Relationship between tumor infiltrating lymphocyte (TIL) levels and response to pembrolizumab (pembro) in metastatic triple-negative breast cancer (mTNBC): results from KEYNOTE-086. Ann Oncol 28:v608

Loi S, Drubay D, Adams S, Pruneri G, Francis PA, Lacroix-Triki M et al (2019) Tumor-infiltrating lymphocytes and prognosis: a pooled individual patient analysis of early-stage triple-negative breast cancers. J Clin Oncol 37(7):559

Loibl S, Untch M, Burchardi N, Huober J, Sinn BV, Blohmer J-U et al (2019) A randomised phase II study investigating durvalumab in addition to an anthracycline taxane-based neoadjuvant therapy in early triple-negative breast cancer: clinical results and biomarker analysis of GeparNuevo study. Ann Oncol 30(8):1279–1288

Luen SJ, Salgado R, Fox S, Savas P, Eng-Wong J, Clark E et al (2017) Tumour-infiltrating lymphocytes in advanced HER2-positive breast cancer treated with pertuzumab or placebo in addition to trastuzumab and docetaxel: a retrospective analysis of the CLEOPATRA study. Lancet Oncol 18(1):52–62

Luen SJ, Salgado R, Dieci MV, Vingiani A, Curigliano G, Gould RE et al (2019) Prognostic implications of residual disease tumor-infiltrating lymphocytes and residual cancer burden in triple-negative breast cancer patients after neoadjuvant chemotherapy. Ann Oncol 30(2):236–242

Mahmoud SMA, Paish EC, Powe DG, Macmillan RD, Grainge MJ, Lee AHS et al (2011) Tumor-infiltrating CD8+ lymphocytes predict clinical outcome in breast cancer. J Clin Oncol 29(15):1949–1955

Mittendorf EΛ, Barrios CH, Harbeck N, Jung KH, Miles D, Saji S et al (2017) IMpassion031: a phase III study comparing neoadjuvant atezolizumab (atezo) vs placebo in combination with anthracycline/nab-paclitaxel (nab-pac)–based chemotherapy in early triple-negative breast cancer (eTNBC). Ann Oncol 28:v65

Mittendorf EA, Zhang H, Barrios CH, Saji S, Jung KH, Hegg R et al (2020) Neoadjuvant atezolizumab in combination with sequential nab-paclitaxel and anthracycline-based chemotherapy versus placebo and chemotherapy in patients with early-stage triple-negative breast cancer (IMpassion031): a randomised, double-blind, phase 3 trial. Lancet 396(10257):1090–1100

Molina R, Auge JM, Farrus B, Zanón G, Pahisa J, Munoz M et al (2010) Prospective evaluation of carcinoembryonic antigen (CEA) and carbohydrate antigen 15.3 (CA 15.3) in patients with primary locoregional breast cancer. Clin Chem 56(7):1148–1157

Müller V, Dieras V, Cardoso F, Cameron D, Cortes J (2021) Expert discussion: highlights from the San Antonio Breast Cancer Symposium, San Antonio, December 8–11, 2020. Breast Care 16(1):89–93. https://www.karger.com/Article/FullText/514333

Nielsen TO, Leung SCY, Rimm DL, Dodson A, Acs B, Badve S et al (2021) Assessment of Ki67 in breast cancer: updated recommendations from the international Ki67 in breast cancer working group. JNCI J Natl Cancer Inst 113(7):808–819

Oh SY, Rahman S, Sparano JA (2021) Perspectives on PARP inhibitors as pharmacotherapeutic strategies for breast cancer. Expert Opin Pharmacother 22(8):981–1003

Oliver J, Quezada Urban R, Franco Cortés CA, Díaz Velásquez CE, Montealegre Paez AL, Pacheco-Orozco RA et al (2019) Latin American study of hereditary breast and ovarian cancer LACAM: a genomic epidemiology approach. Front Oncologia 9:1429

Rebaza P, Calderon G, de la Cruz M, Dunstan J, Cotrina JM, Abugattas J et al (2018) Factores de pronostico en pacientes con cáncer de mama metastásico sometidos a cirugía. Carcinos 8(2):51–60

Rossi G, Mu Z, Rademaker AW, Austin LK, Strickland KS, Costa RLB et al (2018) Cell-free DNA and circulating tumor cells: comprehensive liquid biopsy analysis in advanced breast cancer. Clin Cancer Res 24(3):560–568

Salgado R, Solit DB, Rimm DL, Bogaerts J, Canetta R, Lively T et al (2019) Addressing the dichotomy between individual and societal approaches to personalised medicine in oncology. Eur J Cancer 114:128–136

Schmid P, Adams S, Rugo HS, Schneeweiss A, Barrios CH, Iwata H et al (2018) Atezolizumab and nab-paclitaxel in advanced triple-negative breast cancer. N Engl J Med 379(22):2108–2121

Schmid P, Cortes J, Pusztai L, McArthur H, Kümmel S, Bergh J et al (2020a) Pembrolizumab for early triple-negative breast cancer. N Engl J Med 382(9):810–821

Schmid P, Salgado R, Park YH, Muñoz-Couselo E, Kim SB, Sohn J et al (2020b) Pembrolizumab plus chemotherapy as neoadjuvant treatment of high-risk, early-stage triple-negative breast cancer: results from the phase 1b open-label, multicohort KEYNOTE-173 study. Ann Oncol 31(5):569–581

Sparano JA, Gray RJ, Makower DF, Pritchard KI, Albain KS, Hayes DF et al (2018) Adjuvant chemotherapy guided by a 21-gene expression assay in breast cancer. N Engl J Med 379(2):111–121

Sparano JA, Crager MR, Tang G, Gray RJ, Stemmer SM, Shak S (2021) Development and validation of a tool integrating the 21-gene recurrence score and clinical-pathological features to individualize prognosis and prediction of chemotherapy benefit in early breast cancer. J Clin Oncol 39(6):557–564

Stanton SE, Adams S, Disis ML (2016) Variation in the incidence and magnitude of tumor-infiltrating lymphocytes in breast cancer subtypes: a systematic review. JAMA Oncol 2(10):1354–1360

Voorwerk L, Slagter M, Horlings HM, Sikorska K, van de Vijver KK, de Maaker M et al (2019) Immune induction strategies in metastatic triple-negative breast cancer to enhance the sensitivity to PD-1 blockade: the TONIC trial. Nat Med 25(6):920–928

Wolff AC, Hammond MEH, Allison KH, Harvey BE, Mangu PB, Bartlett JMS et al (2018) Human epidermal growth factor receptor 2 testing in breast cancer: American Society of Clinical Oncology/College of American Pathologists clinical practice guideline focused update. Arch Pathol Lab Med 142(11):1364–1382

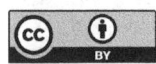

Challenges in Establishing the Clinical Trials Centre at the University of Ulm

Nicole Lang

Challenge: IT Systems

One of the main challenges of the CTC Ulm as joint institution of the Medical Faculty and the University Hospital Ulm is the qualitative and quantitative development of competencies with regard to planning, organisation and conduct of clinical trials to improve translational, patient-oriented research and thus increase study activities according to applicable laws and regulations.

Keys in performing clinical trials are validated, clinical databases that capture, transfer and store data correctly and should comply with current regulatory standards EMA (2020).

Due to the fact that patient's data within a hospital is stored in a secure environment, the data generated in clinical trials also should be stored within this central, protected system. However, the common patient-centred hospital IT system is neither equipped nor prepared for hosting clinical trial data and centrally based data management structures. A dedicated IT team who is trained in clinical trial IT structure requirements and allocated time resource is usually not available. Therefore, the CTC chose relevant clinical trial-related database structures to be hosted externally, which is favourable with regard to the pharmacovigilance database. However, external hosting is not the best option for other relevant data capture systems as the clinical study database (EDC, electronic data capture) due to the high costs of external hosting services and limited flexibility. Therefore, a solution might be to choose a ready-made system including the service of free system installation and minimal regular update and maintenance challenges to the existing IT system.

After identifying about 17 EDC systems, a short review revealed four systems that were not supported anymore and therefore could be excluded. From the remaining 13 systems, 6 were not validated and therefore could be excluded as not providing the needed validation requirements for investigational medicinal product clinical trials. The remaining seven systems were validated EDC systems, but only six of those offered servers within the European Union (EU), which was considered a prerequisite for complying with the legal requirements of the EU General Data Protection Regulation (GDPR). In addition, only four of those six EDC systems offered the possibility of in-house programming of eCRF (electronic case report form) (Fig. 1). The companies providing those remaining EDC

N. Lang (✉)
Medical Faculty and University Hospital of Ulm, Ulm, Germany
e-mail: Nicole.lang@uni-ulm.de

U. Schmidt-Strassburger (ed.), *Improving Oncology Worldwide*, Sustainable Development Goals Series,
https://doi.org/10.1007/978-3-030-96053-7_11

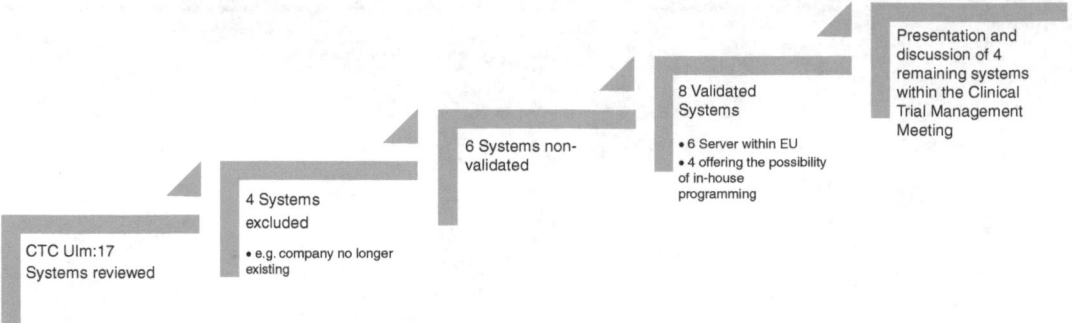

Fig. 1 Review process and numbers of EDC systems screened for suitability for being used within an academic CTC. The figure illustrates the stepwise selection and exclusion process for the identification of an EDC system meeting the requirements (a) to be validated, (b) providing hosting in the EU according to the GDPR and (c) providing eCRFs

systems were invited to present the systems to the university clinical research teams within the Clinical Trial Management Meeting (see section "Governance"). Discussions on costs, hosting systems, flexibility, national user support and availability, as well as familiarity within the academic community, finally lead to a decision for one of these systems.

Establishing a Central Quality Management System

Quality (according to ISO 9000, https://www.iso.org/) is a set of characteristics that a product must have to satisfy needs and expectations of the customer. Indeed, the output (product) from a clinical trial is an information that provides an answer to a scientific question and thus underlies the same standards as any other product.

According to international law and guidelines, one of those being the ICH GCP E6 (R2) (good clinical practice) guideline (https://ichgcp.net/), the sponsor should implement a system to manage quality throughout all stages of the trial process to ensure subject protection and reliability of trial results.

A quality management system (QMS) therefore comprises the design of efficient clinical trial tools and procedures for data collection and processing as well as the control thereof within a quality assurance system.

Quality management consists of quality assurance (QA), comprising all those planned and systematic actions that are established to ensure that the trial is performed and the data are generated, documented, recorded and reported in compliance with GCP and regulatory requirements as SOPs (standard operating procedures) and quality control (QC). QC comprises the operational techniques and activities undertaken within the quality assurance system to verify that the requirements for quality of the trial-related activities have been fulfilled as, for example, monitoring. As within an academic institution as a university and university hospital, the individual clinical trial facilities within the diverse medical specialities generate diverse QMS or parts of it to best comply with required regulation and guidelines. Those decentralised, individual systems provide different quality guidance within SOPs, working instructions as well as QC measures. Therefore, clinical trials, originating from the same sponsor, the University Hospital of Ulm, might range from poor to fair overall quality. To overcome the differing qualities and to guarantee a high-quality standard according to applicable laws and regulations, a centralised QMS for all trials sponsored by the University Hospital Ulm should be implemented, trained and controlled. With a centralised system, insufficient quality within clinical trials and consequential potential harm to patients is more likely ensured to be avoided, and study data integrity is maintained.

The first step within this process is to define and draft overarching, general, central SOPs for clinical trials. This happens with the provision that the major steps are agreed upon by stakeholders, and processes and templates are generated. These SOPs have to be thoroughly taught and made available either through a central platform for clinical trials or a document management system. To assure compliance with these SOPs and general guidance and regulation, and thus adequate quality, major documents of each clinical trial have to undergo a compliance check process within the CTC before sponsor acceptance and signature. In implementing a compliance check that is independent from the clinical trial facility planning the trial, central quality aspects can be implemented for all clinical trials, and GCP compliance can be confirmed. Importantly, the sponsor signature will not be provided without recommendation for signature from the CTC compliance check process, and therefore the compliance check is mandatory for all clinical trials performed at the University Hospital Ulm. Finally, this process leads to a reasonably well-adjusted good quality of all clinical trials performed at the University Hospital Ulm as sponsor of clinical trials. Additionally, the mandatory compliance check task provides a sponsor oversight over existing studies. This oversight is not only requested according to regulation but also needed within other specialities of the Clinical Trials Centre as pharmacovigilance to comply with, for example, cross-reporting obligations.

However, the implementation of a compliance check has to be considered as a first step within the scope of a central QMS for clinical trials. Further quality measures have to be implemented centrally, and compliance should be audited to further improve and control the quality management of clinical trials.

Establishing a Central Pharmacovigilance System

All clinical trials and medical device studies taking place at the University Hospital Ulm (UKU) are subject to the statutory or other provisions to collect, evaluate and report adverse events that occur during the study. SUSARs (suspected unexpected serious adverse reactions) are to be reported electronically to the European EudraVigilance Clinical Trial Module, to ethics committee and to investigators; additionally, a continuous benefit-risk evaluation is mandatory in clinical trials.

As pharmacovigilance requires prompt action and demanding processes in short time frames as well as specially trained pharmacovigilance experts with a proof of work experience in their field, this task was found to be outsourced to CROs (clinical research organisations) at the UKU. A "responsible person for EudraVigilance" must be announced to the EMA (European Medicines Agency), who as a named person represents the sponsor at the European agency and is the point of contact for all safety-related issues for regulatory bodies.

Outsourcing implies several disadvantages in general such as high costs, obscure and complicated processes, the need of controlling and auditing, allocating resources and thus generating redundant processes.

As the Clinical Trials Centre Ulm was faced with the fact that the CRO providing the responsible person function and SUSAR reporting for all IITs (investigator-initiated trials) of the University Hospital Ulm was insolvent, immediate action was necessary. The CTC was notified that services would be stopped within 4 weeks of notification.

Due to this short timeline, a transfer to another CRO including audit, contract negotiations, database and process transfer was not feasible. To guarantee continued safety management for the clinical trials concerned, the CTC decided to assume the responsible person function and SUSAR reporting responsibilities from the CRO. Fortunately, the CTC staff was already trained and listed within the EMA database, and necessary certificates were available.

To guarantee a smooth transition, a central SUSAR reporting email address within UKU was established. Important for choosing this email address was the need to guarantee that external emails, including relevant attachments, will be received in a secure environment (encrypted connection) without being blocked or refuted. In addition, it was indispensable that the CTC staff will be able to access this mailbox 24/7 also from external locations to assure timely processing in accordance with the business continuity plan in case of emergency situations. Additionally, it was guaranteed that this safety email address stored all email conversations and that there is no possibility of emails being deleted or moved by any CTC staff. A regular backup procedure was confirmed to be in place. After successful testing of the email address as well as fax, a process of regular mailbox check was established: The responsible person, deputy or delegates will make sure to regularly check the mailbox for SUSARs according to a predefined schedule, indicating responsibility and backup. It is expected that SUSAR notifications will be sent and received mainly via email, and fax is expected as a fallback solution. Fax will be checked on a daily basis during usual working hours.

After establishing the communication structure at the CTC for SUSAR cases, all stakeholders performing clinical trials had to be identified and notified, and relevant documents of studies concerned had to be amended. All relevant documents (safety management plans, protocols and others) were reviewed for the changes to be implemented due to the pharmacovigilance responsibility transfer from the CRO to the CTC Ulm. Stakeholders were notified by telephone and by email within predefined timelines, and the relevant documents were identified, adapted and signed. Notification dates and acknowledgement dates were tracked within a "CRO-PhV Transfer UKU" table.

To take action according to a predefined strategy and schedule, the transfer modalities and timelines were all documented within a "Transfer Plan." After successful transfer, this "Transfer Plan" was integrated within a "Transfer Document", documenting the transfer and closing the process by signature.

Following this structured approach of process and data transfer, delays or inconsistencies were not noted after the day the system was switched from the CRO to the UKU process, and thus a smooth and successful transition was performed.

By establishing a pharmacovigilance system on-site at the CTC Ulm, streamlined and transparent processes with an adequate price-performance ratio can be set up centrally. Lengthy negotiations with third-party providers are no longer necessary, as are the sometimes complex processes of control and interaction. Pharmacovigilance processes are audit- and inspection-relevant and can be simplified, made transparent and optimised for internal procedures through central SOPs, so that compliance with regulatory requirements is made easier for all those involved. Another advantage is the continuous availability of the expertise on-site, as well as the access to and overview of the safety data at any time, thus guaranteeing the regular risk-benefit assessments required by law.

The sponsorship obligations with regard to pharmacovigilance in IITs are regulated by law. As a sponsor of IITs, the UKU is legally obliged to put in place pharmacovigilance arrangements as sending safety-related information (SUSARs) to the (European/responsible) authority (electronic notification to the EMA (European Medicines Agency)), ethics committee and participating investigators and, if necessary, to data safety monitoring boards (DSMBs)) and marketing authorisation holders (MAHs). The SUSAR reporting to the EMA has to take place centrally via the EudraVigilance database. Pharmacovigilance can be considered a central task per se as the legislation clarifies the ultimate responsibility being with the sponsor of the clinical trial. Therefore, outsourcing to a CRO has different implications as on the one hand being costly, and cost considerations are always high priority within the public sector. On the other hand, due to the sponsor obligations as outlined above, extensive oversight mechanism of third-party providers would have to be established, which would lead to resource allocation at the sponsor site. After review of existing processes with CROs, we found extensive, intransparent, time-consuming and error-prone processes, resulting in potential incompliance with pharmacovigilance legal and regulatory requirements. In accordance with Dinnett et al. (2013), we concluded that without a centralised pharmacovigilance system, the pharmacovigilance responsibilities of the sponsor are hardly to be adequately fulfilled.

Therefore, in order to meet the legal requirements for drug safety in the studies initiated at the UKU (IIT), as well as to provide the qualitative requirements to guarantee a high level of patient safety and regulatory compliance, streamlined processes and development of know-how and cross-departmental specialist expertise in pharmacovigilance locally, it was decided to implement a centralised pharmacovigilance system within the UKU. To meet these requirements, a GCP-compliant pharmacovigilance database (PhV-DB), and a pharmacovigilance quality management system (PhV QMS), including training of its management has to be implemented.

The refinancing of the pharmacovigilance system to be established at the CTC takes place through an internally defined scale of fees and represents a cost-adapted solution to the situation of self-initiated medical research in university medicine.

The goal of providing a pharmacovigilance system with a high-quality pharmacovigilance database that meets current regulatory requirements, embedded in a pharmacovigilance QMS for self-initiated studies at the UKU, represents a major local advantage for medical research at the University of Ulm (Table 1).

With regard to IT (information technology) resource limitations as well as limited knowledge in validation procedures, an in-house solution with a self-developed pharmacovigilance DB was found to be unfeasible due to the extensive regulatory requirements of the pharmacovigilance database. Therefore, it was decided to approach PhV database vendors for feasible solutions.

Before screening PhV database vendors, intensive communications and discussion with the stakeholders of the individual study centres were performed. Information about the current pharmacovigilance solutions (status quo) and processes was obtained. A needs analysis as well

Table 1 Advantages and challenges of a central pharmacovigilance (PhV) system at the UKU

Advantages	Challenges
Development of internal know-how and cross-departmental specialist expertise	Liability to keep up to date with (inter-)national regulations and guidelines, responsibility to create a robust education and training system
Independence from external service providers	Responsibility for maintaining an internal robust PhV system including specific PhV staff who will serve as PhV team and office space
Streamlined and effective processes, easy to adapt	May be viewed as another internal bureaucratic burden for investigators and clinical trial staff
Ensuring a high quality of the data through a validated pharmacovigilance database and uniform, standardised data entry and quality standards as well as processes	Purchasing a validated electronic secure central pharmacovigilance database conforming to international requirements of electronic submission of safety reports[a]
Development of a PhV QMS and continuous adaptation to the needs of medical research at the University of Ulm	Establishing standard processes translated into standard operating procedures (SOPs) that have to be reviewed and adapted regularly
Attractive price solution through internal service (no VAT, no overhead)	Risk of increased costs during decreased PhV needs
Cost-effective	Risk of maintaining PhV staff and offices during decreased amount of PhV activity
Resources saved by saving tenders, contract negotiations and lengthy communication with service providers	Not applicable
Resources saved by saving audits at service providers (CRO) and extensive oversight mechanisms	Not applicable
Guarantee of regulatory compliance through internal, centrally valid SOPs	Building and achieving a system acceptable and compliant to any auditor and inspector

[a] ICH guideline E2B (R3) on electronic transmission of individual case safety reports (ICSRs)—data elements and message specification—implementation guide

as a query of needed capacities regarding the provision of study-specific pharmacovigilance services at the UKU was performed. Analysis of the findings revealed the volume of cases and required processes so that vendors of two PhV databases were approached and compared with regard to price, support services, follow-up costs and expenses (e.g. required in-house validation), server location, validation (GAMP-5), MedDRA implementation, guaranteed availability time, gateway function to EMA, etc. Other CTCs using these databases were interviewed and pros and cons opposed. Finally, a decision for one of the systems was made during a CTC board meeting.

Subsequently, the CTC Ulm began with the creation and implementation of a PhV QMS (SOPs, manuals, conventions) and subsequent training of the employees of the study centres as well as information of the respective clinics, institutes and project managers.

The pharmacovigilance system consisting of the pharmacovigilance database and the PhV QMS, which in addition to SOPs, manuals, conventions and other documents also includes the necessary training for internal employees, project managers and collaborators as well as study participants, is being developed and continuously adapted by the CTC Ulm.

Objectives of the implementation of a central pharmacovigilance system at the CTC are the following:

1. Support of medical research and relief of the study centres by creating ICSRs (individual case safety reports) and other necessary reports (including DSURs/SAE listings) on adverse events from clinical trials.
2. Provision of a high-quality pharmacovigilance standard through a pharmacovigilance system for the documentation and tracking of serious adverse events (e.g. for DSMBs) as well as reporting of SUSARs to the EMA and respective competent authorities nationally and internationally according to legal requirements (mandatory electronically via EMA portal from CTC Ulm). This also includes the

creation of data sets that are consistent and complete in terms of content, which can be sent to all institutions/affected persons within the narrow legally prescribed time window, thus promoting and ensuring the contemporary and required quality of clinical trials in the field of pharmacovigilance.
3. Promotion and implementation of a uniform and high-quality procedure within the UKU with regard to SAE processing and data entry through the provision of central SOPs, data entry and coding conventions, as well as regular training (PhV QMS).

Central Training

As part of a university medicine medical faculty and central structure of clinical trial research, a CTC is responsible for training and further educating employees involved in clinical studies for their special requirements. Training is a cornerstone to enable investigators and study staff to conduct clinical trials safely and ensure the implementation of clinical studies according to applicable laws and guidelines. Training and advanced training are therefore essential aspects of a CTC. In order to meet these requirements, the CTCs, which are part of the CTC network (KKS-Netzwerk e. V. n.d.), have established their own departments, which guarantee high-quality training and further education of qualified study staff for the implementation of clinical studies as well as for the further training of medical professionals in the field of study design and coordination (Stellungnahme der Arbeitsgruppe "Klinische Studien" der DFG-Senatskommission für Grundsatzfragen in der Klinischen Forschung 2018; Wissenschaftsrat 2018).

The training courses include ethical, regulatory, qualitative, safety, operational and other scientific requirements for clinical studies in order to ensure the implementation according to global quality and safety standards. The qualification and training of study staff ensure the safety of the study participants on-site and the validity and robustness of the study data.

Depending on the course programme, the CTC organises the certification of the courses by the German Medical Association and approval by the ethics committee. The medical participants receive appropriate training points (CME) from the medical association after successfully passing a knowledge test. The courses are continuously evaluated by the participants as well as the training management and adjusted accordingly.

The challenges of implementing such a central training environment are organisational as well as content related. With regard to organisational aspects, the following issues need to be considered: A lecture room or an auditorium for up to 150 participants needs to be reserved. As some trainings are whole-day trainings or even comprise several days, catering should be offered. Upfront, invitations, agenda and further information and communication should be disseminated. The target audience has to be defined, and the means of communication such as email, publication within print media or within intra- and/or Internet page has to be determined. For drafting a participation list, registration should be organised by a predefined central email address and contact, and each registration should be followed by registration approval message. If the training is held by live webinar, the system and webinar platform needs to be tested upfront; in general, IT support should be organised before and during the whole meeting to resolve upcoming issues with login and connection. In general, automatic functions as training registration approval message should be considered. After the training, tests need to be collected and reviewed. A process for failed participants and the possibility of re-testing should be defined upfront. Confirmation of participation and training certificates need to be printed, signed and forwarded to the participants. Finally, the evaluation sheets need to be reviewed and possible actions taken.

With regard to organisational aspects, an early start should be envisaged, and the efforts should not be underestimated. Therefore, enough time should be reserved for the preparation as well as follow-up activities.

With regard to content-related aspects, experts within their fields need to be identified and asked for their willingness to prepare and hold a lecture as part of the training. Backup solutions should be in place for individuals, and the presentations need to be collected upfront and reviewed by the study team for content and format.

The challenge of training and transfer of study-related knowledge as, for example, GCP to all stakeholders in all parts of the academic research facilities is a key part of quality assurance in clinical studies.

Governance

It is key to implement a central, superordinate institution for implementing overarching standards for clinical trials according to applicable laws, regulations and guidelines, GCP as well as local processes. As the sponsor oversight needs to be guaranteed by law, it was decided that stakeholders at the individual study centres should be identified and invited to regular meetings for information exchange. This meeting was named Clinical Trial Management (CTM) meeting and invites all stakeholders not only to be informed about the current status and standards of clinical studies at the UKU but also to be actively involved in decisions and upcoming actions. To be invited to the CTM meeting, the CTC asks within the introductory visit at the clinics and institutes for a representative and deputy to be invited to regular CTM meetings. These stakeholders are the links to the individual study centres in the different departments and responsible for disseminating the information provided within the CTM meetings. Also, dedicated project groups, which concentrate on specific solutions, are recruited from the CTM members and report their solutions to the CTM team. Based on these meetings, governance was implemented and is executed by the CTC.

References

Dinnett et al (2013) Implementing a centralised pharma-covigilance service in a non-commercial setting in the United Kingdom Trials. 14:171.

EMA (2020) Notice to sponsors on validation and qualification of computerised systems used in clinical trials. EU Regulation 536/2014, FDA Title 21 CRF Part 11, ICH E6.

KKS-Netzwerk e. V. (n.d.). https://www.kks-netzwerk.de/index.php

Stellungnahme der Arbeitsgruppe "Klinische Studien" der DFG-Senatskommission für Grundsatzfragen in der Klinischen Forschung. Bonn, 2018.

Wissenschaftsrat. Empfehlungen zu Klinischen Studien. Drs. 7301–18 Hannover 19 10 2018.

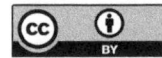

Improving Patient Care

Patriciu-Andrei Achimaş-Cadariu

Cancer Burden

Due to higher life expectancy and drastic lifestyle changes, the burden of cancer is rising in low- and middle-income countries (LMICs) and is becoming an alarming public health issue (Shah et al. 2019). Disparities and inequities in healthcare access, poor education and public health policies with no preventive strategies, high cost of treatment and deprioritization of non-communicable diseases (NCDs), including cancers, are significant issues. The economic impact of premature mortality due to neoplasia, increased morbidity and low budget allocations for health also stresses an already weakened healthcare system that is not sustainable. Strengthening aspects such as education on health and lifestyle can alleviate primary prevention of neoplasia. Vaccination programmes for infectious agents such as HBV and HPV can successfully reduce cancer burden (Hussein et al. 2016), while screening programmes increase early detection of neoplasia as part of secondary prevention. Such strategies require universal healthcare access through alleviating the cost for the population, decentralization of screening and diagnosis centres and

P.-A. Achimaş-Cadariu (✉)
Iuliu Hatieganu University of Medicine and Pharmacy, Cluj-Napoca, Romania

Ion Chiricuta Institute of Oncology, Cluj-Napoca, Romania

proper funding. Such policies can only be sustainable if proper treatment is given following every irregularity found in screening programmes. Facilities for cancer treatment are usually scattered in LMICs. However, resources should be made available to the population through outreach programmes, universal health insurance, collaborations with high-income countries (HICs), in parallel with infrastructure development, multidisciplinary management of oncological patients and cancer research. Supportive and survivorship care, together with palliative care, are critical and should be implemented whenever possible.

Surgical Oncology

Optimizing cancer care and surgical oncology is a crucial milestone in the integrative care of oncological patients. Surgery is essential for cancer treatment globally, but less than 25% of patients with cancer worldwide get safe, affordable or timely surgery (Sullivan et al. 2015). There have been reported wide equity gaps, and patients from rural LMIC areas are particularly at risk for lack of access to surgery, often because of economic constraints and lack of service (Sullivan et al. 2015). Considering that surgery is cost-effective and, if applied in locally confined tumours, curative, the current situation will widen the service gap instead of achieving the

U. Schmidt-Strassburger (ed.), *Improving Oncology Worldwide*, Sustainable Development Goals Series, https://doi.org/10.1007/978-3-030-96053-7_12

Sustainable Development Goal (SDG) Target 3.4 ("By 2030, reduce by one third premature mortality from non-communicable diseases through prevention and treatment and promote mental health and well-being") because of missing SDG Target 3.8 ("Achieve universal health coverage, including financial risk protection, access to quality essential health-care services and access to safe, effective, quality and affordable essential medicines and vaccines for all").

India is the second largest country by population, and more than 70% of its population lives in rural areas with scarce resources, education and health access. In addition to disparities in healthcare access, for 2018, cancer incidence in India was estimated at more than 1.1 million new cases with an extremely high mortality to incidence ratio (Dhillon et al. 2018). Moreover, there is no central accreditation board for surgical oncology. As a result, cancer treatment facilities, already weak in infrastructure, are overcrowded, while poorly trained doctors treat patients. The cost of treatment is also extremely high due to high rates of privatization and poor social and health insurance policies, thus forcing patients to give up treatment sometimes. It is estimated that 80% of oncological patients will need surgery, making timely, optimal and affordable surgery a priority in cancer care (Sullivan et al. 2015). Steps in the right direction have been made with the implementation of the National Cancer Grid (NCG) that aims to supervise cancer care (Pramesh et al. 2014), injecting capital into healthcare with increases as high as 137% more than in previous years and through the National Programme for Prevention and Control of Cancer, Diabetes, Cardiovascular Diseases and Stroke (NPCDCS).

Palliative Care

As life expectancy improves worldwide, there is also a growing need for palliative care integrated with preventive medicine, early diagnosis and optimal treatment (Palliative Care 2021). Palliative care is the multidisciplinary practice that improves the quality of life amongst patients (both adults and children) and their families who are facing issues related to a chronic or terminal illness; these may include but are not limited to identification and treatment of pain, physical, spiritual or psychosocial challenges. Early-stage symptom control is an ethical duty, and palliation is the most effective if applied early on. It reduces unnecessary hospital admissions while relieving suffering and offering dignity to patients. Health systems are responsible at a national level to include palliative care in the routine care of terminally ill or chronic patients. It is estimated that 40 million people worldwide require palliative services, while 78% live in LMIC countries. Unfortunately, only 14% of people in need of palliation receive appropriate services. This is primarily due to the lack of awareness among policymakers, inadequate funding, cultural and social barriers and perhaps unnecessarily restrictive regulations for palliative medicines. While subspeciality palliative care is a stand-alone medical speciality in many HICs, primary palliative care can be integrated at all the levels of a healthcare system even by practitioners with no former training in such practices. These services may include pain management or other physical symptoms by primary usage of pain medication, routine care of patients and care coordination. Primary palliation must be provided early on, alleviating pain and suffering and reducing care fragmentation in an empathic manner.

Iran has a population of more than 82 million. The current prevalence of cancer in Iran is more than 300,000 cases, and more than 100,000 patients add to these numbers annually. The need for palliation is palpable. While still in its infancy, palliative care in Iran can be an example of good practice. Modern practices date back to 2000 when experts in Iran collaborated with the Royal Hospital for Women in Australia and the Sydney Institute of Palliative Medicine. Training in palliative care started in the Cancer Research Center in Tehran back in 2006, while integrating palliative subspeciality training into clinical practice was established through a palliative medicine fellowship programme in 2012. One or two palliative care specialists graduate each year; however, palliation in Iran is still not well structured. This is due to a disorganized system, a shortage of trained specialists and the deprioritization of NCDs in the face of the COVID-19 pandemic. The current initiative, involving the help of the University of Ulm, Germany, and the Center for Palliative Medicine at the University Hospital of Cologne, Germany, strives to create an online educational platform in Farsi language to aid palliative care in Iran.

Paediatric Oncology

Paediatric oncology represents another challenge in integrated cancer care. HICs report over 80% survival rates for patients with paediatric neoplasias, whereas those in LMICs average at about 20% (Childhood Cancer 2021). Even though cancers are comparatively rare in children compared to cancers in adults (Cancer Statistics 2021), the burden on affected families and their grief and mental health is not to be underestimated. It is, therefore, necessary to seek solutions for the most vulnerable of society. Knowledge transfer from HICs to LMICs is desirable for strengthening collaborations and establishing a sustainable scientific exchange.

Armenia is the perfect example that succeeded in overcoming the unmet needs of children with cancer. In 1994, the survival rate of children with acute lymphocytic leukaemia (ALL) was 0.7%, while in 2019, it was 73.3% after implementing standardized protocols (Krmoyan et al. 2019). Good practices were disseminated through collaborations with cancer centres in the USA, Germany, Taiwan, Austria and Belgium. Collective efforts founded the Armenian Association of Hematology and Oncology (AAHO), created a united Pediatric Cancer and Blood Disorders Center of Armenia (PCBDCA), only to start, in 2019, a three-year fellowship for paediatric haematology-oncology. While having to overcome issues like the government not subsidizing some cancer treatments, Armenia proved that LMICs could meet the needs of paediatric cancer patients with the help of and through collaborative projects with HICs.

Quality Assurance in Oncology

The administration of procedures like chemotherapy, radiation therapy, surgery and all imaging modalities happens with the provision that these are safe. Analyses by one of the leading scientific societies in oncology have shown that adherence to standards is less stringent the longer a physician practises her/his speciality (Blayney et al. 2020). Moreover, quality control should be carried out regularly to ensure optimal care for all cancer patients. The American Society of Clinical Oncology (ASCO) developed a quality programme called the Quality Oncology Practice Initiative (QOPI), wich has been open for worldwide registration since 2016 (Blayney et al. 2020). Such programmes warrant a proper assessment of patients and ensure high-quality outpatient practices with the aim of constant self-actualization of the treatment team and the applied pathways. With oncology as a rapidly evolving discipline, this self-actualization is essential for providing services that meet the patients' und the physicians' highest standards while ensuring organizational and financial safety and thus sustainability.

A group of practising oncologists in Brazil officially obtained the QOPI Certification Program (QCP) accreditation in February 2020 and is an eloquent example that implementing quality cancer care at international standards can be feasible in more places. This experience will be described in the chapter "Quality Oncology Practice Improvement (QOPI) in Brazil: A Successful Knowledge Transfer Under the Auspices of the American Society of Clinical Oncology (ASCO)".

Comprehensive Cancer Centres

Through the centuries, cancer centres have evolved in places with high incidence, subsequently becoming also research facilities. The cancer centre I am directing was founded over 90 years ago and had already incorporated an epidemiological approach to oncology thereby paving the way to possible treatments of these ailments. In France, cancer centres integrating basic research were founded after World War II, and in the USA, the National Cancer Act of 1971 led to the foundation of cancer centres and, subsequently, the Comprehensive Cancer Centres (CCCs).

Research, education and outreach and multidisciplinary management are significant features of a Comprehensive Cancer Centre (CCC), as a model borrowed from the USA, currently adopted by other countries like Germany (Comprehensive Cancer Center Ulm (CCCU) | Universitätsklinikum Ulm 2021). CCCs are expected to conduct and initiate clinical trials, sustain basic and translational research and provide quality management of such activities. Tumour boards with regular meetings should give recommendations for every patient, while multidisciplinary teams provide timely, optimal and affordable state-of-the-art cancer management. Therefore, many challenges arise while running a CCC, including but not limited to providing adequate infrastructure that can sustain all of the requirements above, funding, finding an optimal quality management system that can ensure proper adherence to international quality standards, outreach programmes, palliative care and many more.

COVID-19-Related Service Disruption

One of the most recent struggles for healthcare systems worldwide is the COVID-19 pandemic. While the first cases were recorded in 2019 in Wuhan City, China, the disease spread easily and was characterized quickly as a pandemic (Coronavirus disease (COVID-19) – World Health Organization 2021), taking by surprise even the most prepared healthcare systems, now having to face a new disease, with no evidence-based treatment with a shortage of protective gear, ICU beds and ventilators. Quick reallocation of human, logistic and financial resources towards a new crisis meant that NCDs were no longer a priority. Therefore, many preventive programmes for neoplasia were deferred, slowing down or coming to a complete halt (Richards et al. 2020). Meanwhile, government officials issued many restrictions, including lockdowns and sanitary measures that, together with natural immunization and later on

through vaccination, led to a decrease of the COVID-19 disease burden. Various resources became available for physicians worldwide in hopes of aiding medical specialists in staying up to date with the latest medical news, such as www.howitreatcovid19.com (How I Treat COVID-19 | Management of the COVID-19 Pandemic 2021). However, slowly restarting screening programmes brought up a new challenge in the form of excess diagnosis (Jones et al. 2020; Yong et al. 2020; Marine et al. 2020).

It became quickly apparent that harvesting the COVID-19 momentum is a fundamental turning point moving forward in most healthcare systems and public health policies worldwide. Appropriate simulation models can estimate optimal catching-up strategies for mitigating the deferred preventive services (Creating et al. 2021; Castanon et al. 2021a,b) while evaluating the feasibility of deploying different models like age-related risk stratification (Castanon et al. 2021a), since triaging and prioritizing patients is a must moving forward. As healthcare systems proved to be very reactive to change, some strategies seem like they are here to stay, like telemedicine and other uses of technology such as self-sampling for HPV. Vaccination facilities worldwide can be further capitalized on for HBV or HPV vaccination, borrowing strategies previously used in the COVID-19 pandemic such as vaccination marathons and intensive media coverage with proper funding and guidance. Elective surgery should be restarted responsibly (*Anaesthesia* 2021) as further challenges such as providing COVID-19-free pathways for NCDs, cancers included, arise.

To summarize, NCDs, neoplasias included, have a considerable impact on all levels of society. Cancer patients should not be neglected despite the current epidemiological, financial or logistical challenges a healthcare system faces, while timely, affordable and safe cancer management should always be provided.

References

(2021) Timing of surgery following SARS-CoV-2 infection: an international prospective cohort study. Anaesthesia 76(6):748–758. https://doi.org/10.1111/anae.15458

Blayney D, Albdelhafeez N, Jazieh A et al (2020) International perspective on the pursuit of quality in cancer care: global application of QOPI and QOPI certification. J Glob Oncol 6:697–703. https://doi.org/10.1200/go.20.00048

Cancer Statistics (2021) National Cancer Institute. https://www.cancer.gov/about-cancer/understanding/statistics. Accessed 6 June 2021

Castanon A, Rebolj M, Burger E et al (2021a) Cervical screening during the COVID-19 pandemic: optimizing recovery strategies. Lancet Public Health 6(7):e522–e527. https://doi.org/10.1016/s2468-2667(21)00078-5

Castanon A, Rebolj M, Pesola F, Sasieni P (2021b) Recovery strategies following COVID-19 disruption to cervical cancer screening and their impact on excess diagnoses. Br J Cancer 124(8):1361–1365. https://doi.org/10.1038/s41416-021-01275-3

Childhood Cancer (2021) Who.int. https://www.who.int/news-room/fact-sheets/detail/cancer-in-children. Accessed 7 June 2021

Comprehensive Cancer Center Ulm (CCCU) | Universitätsklinikum Ulm (2021) Uniklinik-ulm.de. https://www.uniklinik-ulm.de/comprehensive-cancer-center-ulm-cccu.html. Accessed 7 June 2021

Coronavirusdisease(COVID-19)–WorldHealthOrganization (2021) Who.int. https://www.who.int/emergencies/diseases/novel-coronavirus-2019?gclid=Cj0KCQjwh_eFBhDZARIsALHjIKeAx_4acFUCB-dJ53xU-5giz2t2uhGvpTlWlI0_d5ZTJPztfHKMya4aAq8eE-ALw_wcB. Accessed 7 June 2021

Creating L, Kaljouw S, de Jonge L et al (2021) Effects of cancer screening restart strategies after COVID-19 disruption. Br J Cancer 124(9):1516–1523. https://doi.org/10.1038/s41416-021-01261-9

Dhillon P, Mathur P, Nandakumar A et al (2018) The burden of cancers and their variations across the states of India: the global burden of disease study 1990–2016. Lancet Oncol 19(10):1289–1306. https://doi.org/10.1016/s1470-2045(18)30447-9

How I Treat COVID-19 | Management of the COVID-19 Pandemic (2021) How I Treat COVID-19. https://howitreatcovid19.com/. Accessed 7 June 2021

Hussein W, Anwar W, Attaleb M et al (2016) A review of the infection-associated cancers in North African countries. Infect Agent Cancer 11(1). https://doi.org/10.1186/s13027-016-0083-8

Jones D, Neal R, Duffy S, Scott S, Whitaker K, Brain K (2020) Impact of the COVID-19 pandemic on the symptomatic diagnosis of cancer: the view from primary care. Lancet Oncol 21(6):748–750. https://doi.org/10.1016/s1470-2045(20)30242-4

Krmoyan L, Danielyan S, Tamamyan G et al (2019) Childhood acute Leukemias in Armenia. Clin Lymph Myel Leuke 19:S195. https://doi.org/10.1016/j.clml.2019.07.043

Marine C, Spicer J, Morris M et al (2020) The impact of the COVID-19 pandemic on cancer deaths due to delays in diagnosis in England, UK: a national, population-based, modelling study. Lancet Oncol 21(8):1023–1034. https://doi.org/10.1016/s1470-2045(20)30388-0

Palliative Care (2021) Who.int. https://www.who.int/health-topics/palliative-care. Accessed 7 June 2021

Pramesh C, Badwe R, Sinha R (2014) The National Cancer Grid of India. Indian J Med Paediatr Oncol 35(3):226. https://doi.org/10.4103/0971-5851.142040

Richards M, Anderson M, Carter P, Ebert B, Mossialos E (2020) The impact of the COVID-19 pandemic on cancer care. Nat Cancer 1(6):565–567. https://doi.org/10.1038/s43018-020-0074-y

Shah S, Kayamba V, Peek R, Heimburger D (2019) Cancer control in low- and middle-income countries: is it time to consider screening? J Glob Oncol 5:1–8. https://doi.org/10.1200/jgo.18.00200

Sullivan R, Alatise O, Anderson B et al (2015) Global cancer surgery: delivering safe, affordable, and timely cancer surgery. Lancet Oncol 16(11):1193–1224. https://doi.org/10.1016/s1470-2045(15)00223-5

Yong J, Mainprize J, Yaffe M et al (2020) The impact of episodic screening interruption: COVID-19 and population-based cancer screening in Canada. J Med Screen 28(2):100–107. https://doi.org/10.1177/0969141320974711

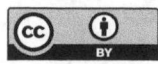

Essential Elements in Improving Oncology in Low- and Middle-Income Countries (LMICs) and Examples for Their Implementation in Nigeria

Atara Ntekim

Introduction

The burden of cancer is increasing in LMICs due to higher life expectancy, westernization of lifestyle, and reduced childhood mortality (El Saghir et al. 2014). This is a source of great public health concern. There is poor uptake and implementation of preventive measures as well as poor access to early diagnosis and treatment. Together, these lead to a high proportion of patients presenting with advanced diseases. Outcomes of cancer treatment correlate with the degree of early detection and diagnostic efficiency paired with appropriate and timely management. Other factors that contribute to the poor outlook of cancer in LMICs include a lower level of education and awareness in lay and health-care communities, poor public awareness and information on cancer, poverty, weak health-care system, and death of cancer health-care personnel. There is also poor research output on preventive, diagnostic, and interventional methods relevant to the population taking into consideration, appropriate methods, and technology in fighting cancer. The aim of this chapter is to highlight essential elements needed to prevent cancer and improve care of cancer patients in LMICs.

A. Ntekim (✉)
Department of Radiation Oncology, College of Medicine, University of Ibadan Nigeria, Ibadan, Nigeria

Prevention and Early Detection

The problem: Certain habits and lifestyles are known to predispose to some cancers. These include tobacco and alcohol use, intake of fatty foods, sedentary lifestyle, and obesity (Katzke et al. 2015). Reduction in the indulgence with these habits and lifestyles as well as control of obesity are essential as measures of primary prevention of cancer. Tobacco smoking is an important risk factor for cancers, especially cancers of lung, head, and neck region and esophagus and bladder cancer (El Saghir et al. 2014). More people in LMICs indulge in tobacco smoking more than before as a sign of new wealth or as part of westernized lifestyle (Editors The Lancet Respiratory Medicine 2019). Education and anti-smoking legislation/campaigns are relatively weak in LMICs. Strengthening these aspects including restricting smoking in public places and screen adverts on tobacco can reduce smoking habits especially among adolescents and young adults. Dietary factors are responsible for about 20% of cancers in LMICs (El Saghir et al. 2014). These can be reduced through intense and sustained public education on promoting healthy diets and increased physical activity as well as proper food storage.

Possible solutions: Education on healthy food habits and lifestyles starting in kindergartens, schools, and throughout all mass media can raise public awareness and introduce behavioral changes

U. Schmidt-Strassburger (ed.), *Improving Oncology Worldwide*, Sustainable Development Goals Series, https://doi.org/10.1007/978-3-030-96053-7_13

that will ultimately lead to the adoption of healthier habits. Alcohol and tobacco abuse education and tobacco cessation programs can help to drop these habits together with stress management programs for all ages and physical education.

In Nigeria, efforts are being made to enlighten the public on the need for healthy habits and life-styles, but these efforts are sporadic and—so far—not consistent. Furthermore, such activities concentrate on cities and urban areas whereas the rural areas, where about 80% of the population live, are hardly reached. Primary prevention and education require more funding to be provided to support nationwide enlightenment campaigns on healthy living.

Control of Infections Associated with Cancer

The problem: Close to 30% of cancers in LMICs are associated with infections (Shah et al. 2019). The control of the spread of these infective agents constitutes a part of primary prevention of cancer. Notably among these infective agents are human papilloma virus (HPV), which is associated with the development of cervical cancer, and hepatitis B virus (HBV), which is associated with the development of hepatocellular carcinoma (Hussein et al. 2016). Even though effective vac-cines are available for the prevention of these two infections, the uptake and coverage for these vac-cinations are still low in LMICs. These are partly due to the lack of sustainable vaccination pro-grams that enable eligible individuals free access to the vaccines and the lack of financial capacity for individuals to pay for the vaccines. The high prevalence of human immunodeficiency virus (HIV) in many LMICs is also a factor responsible for the high incidence of HIV-associated cancers in these countries. People living with HIV are vulnerable to AIDS-associated malignancies and other malignancies with poor treatment outcomes.

Possible solutions are prevention education, sex education starting in kindergarten and schools, empowering women econonomically, vaccination programs with widespread media coverage, and destigmatization of people living with HIV and cancer. In Nigeria, the coverage of HPV and HBV vaccination is quite low. This is largely due to poor access due to cost. The price reduction of HBV and HPV vaccines will greatly contribute to an increase in the uptake of the vac-cine in LMICs. In addition, public education and campaigning on the usefulness of vaccination should be stepped up to improve uptake and sup-port of vaccination programs.

HIV treatment is better because there were international donors that supported the diagnosis and treatment. Such aids are needed to make HPV and HBV vaccinations available to a larger population. Current efforts toward the control of HIV infections should be strengthened and sus-tained to reduce the incidence and morbidity associated with HIV infection to enlist a reduc-tion in HIV-associated cancers.

Improving Cancer Screening and Diagnosis

The problem: Cancer screening has been reported to contribute significantly to the low cancer-related mortality in high-income countries (HICs) (Sankaranarayanan 2014). This is particularly true for cervical, breast, and colorectal cancers. Screening programs are nonexistent in most LMICs, and where available, they are at great cost and therefore not affordable by most patients, who pay out of pocket for these services. In addi-tion to these, screening facilities are scanty and not close to where most people reside.

Possible solutions: Efforts towards the reduc-tion of cost especially for the most prevalent can-cers, namely, breast, cervical, prostate, and colorectal cancers, will improve uptake of screen-ing tests thereby leading to early diagnosis and effective treatment. These cost reductions should be communicated together with the health bene-fits of the respective screening programs.

In Nigeria, there is no established program for cancer screening. Individuals pay for their screen-ing, and screening centers are also not readily available as they are mostly located in tertiary hospitals. Primary health-care facilities should be adequately prepared to take part in some aspects of screening such as taking samples in the case of cervical cancer screening and shipping them to the closest tertiary centers for processing and analysis. Mobile mammography vans and boats should be procured to visit primary health-care centers in remote areas including riverine communities at intervals to conduct screenings at subsidized rates. Clinical teams can also visit primary health-care centers at intervals to carry out screening activities and counseling.

Availability of Diagnostic Methods

The problem: Diagnosis plays an important role in the prevention and treatment of cancer. Communities with low-quality diagnostic infrastructure will underreport the cancer burden in their areas (Cazap et al. 2016). In most LMICs, diagnostic facilities are poor and most of them are in urban centers.

Possible solutions: The assessment of cancer burden in communities requires both the training of personnel and availability of equipment to provide these services. In particular, diagnostic facilities will improve cancer diagnosis and treatment.

In Nigeria, as an interim measure, centrally located diagnostic centers with optimal facilities could be established in districts, and samples could be collected and sent to such centers for analysis. With the availability of courier services and other means of transport and communication, samples could be transported to such centers and results sent to the requesting health-care facilities by secured emails or text messages. This arrangement could also be used for investigations such as genetic/genomic profiles that cannot be done in-country presently.

Optimizing Patient Management

The problem: Access to care is limited in LMICs. This is due to lack of enough cancer care facilities (Haier et al. 2019). Radiation therapy is an important modality of cancer treatment, and it contributes to the cure or palliation. About 50%

of cancer patients will require radiation treatment at one time or the other during the course of their cancer care (Delaney et al. 2005). In Nigeria as in other LMICs, the availability of radiotherapy facilities is less than one machine to one million people compared with more than five machines to one million people in a developed country like Canada according to IAEA DIRAC database (Fig. 1) (IAEA 2021).

So far, facilities for cancer treatment are too few in LMICs, and where they are available, the cost is high. The various stages of cancer management, namely, diagnosis, staging, treatment, follow-up, and palliative care, require physicians who specialize in these aspects. According to a recent IAEA (International Atomic Energy Agency) report, there is a shortage of about 50,000 cancer care professionals in developing countries necessitating the need for institutions in the developed world to collaborate toward training of manpower for LMICs (IAEA 2020). These specialists are therefore few in most LMICs. In some instances, they may not be available. Early detection requires appropriate treatment for good disease control. Many patients travel far distances to access care, which is associated with high cost for them. Many of the patients cannot afford the financial demands needed to access care and therefore abandoned treatment at various stages.

Possible solutions: Introduction of universal health insurance to cover cancer services and generating funds to subsidize cancer treatments would substantially improve the uptake of services. Many governments and philanthropists can improve the uptake of complete cancer services. In addition, it will be in the interest of the entire population to create own sickness funds based on principles of solidarity and that every employer should contribute to these sickness funds.

Hostels with less expensive accommodation may offer their services near major cancer treatment centers to ease problems associated with lodging away from home to access treatment. Primary care must be made available through establishment of cancer centers in regions closer to the people. Outreach programs organized to reach rural populations may include some aspects of cancer services.

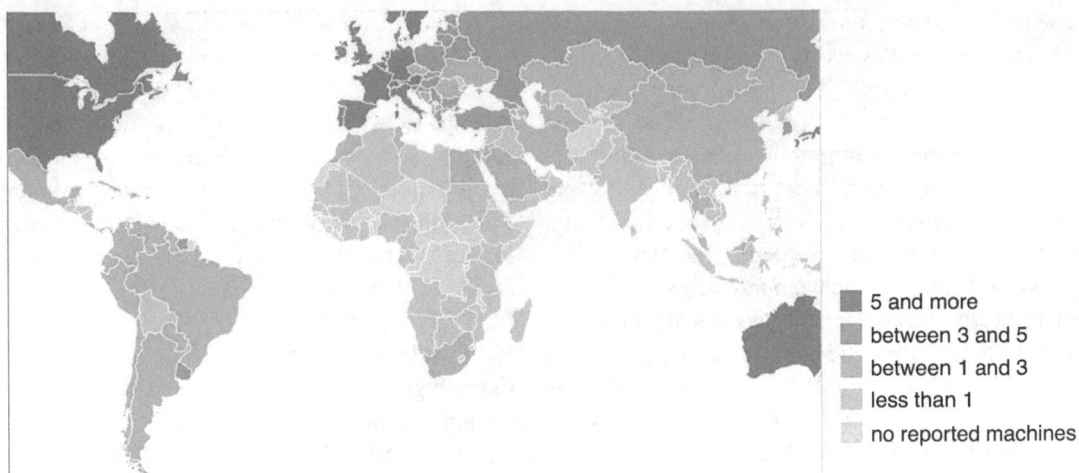

Fig. 1 Number of radiotherapy machines per million people (Source: IAEA Directory of Radiotherapy Centers (DIRAC) (IAEA 2021)

Following the diagnosis of cancer, resources should be available to address the treatment of the patient with the identified disease. Collaboration with HICs to support cancer care services through donations and other supports is important if services cannot—yet—be provided by the home country of the patient. There could also be a joint review of investigation results and management plans of patients between healthcare professionals in LMICs and HICs, as shown in the Cure4Kids initiative by St. Jude Children's Research Hospital (https://www.cure4kids.org/) in the USA or the Mayo and Cleveland Clinic outreach programs. These can be Internet-based to ensure optimal treatment and exchange between highly qualified professionals.

Research

1. Cancer research provides the way through which cancer care improved in HICs (Barrios et al. 2018). Through research, effective methods of diagnosis and treatment relevant to the population are being identified, developed, and put into practice.

   The problem: There is a low level of research in most LMICs. Little is budgeted for research leading to a low impact of research on cancer care. Research activities covering the assessment of the current status of cancer incidence (registries), clinical research with a focus on the population served, and behavioral research for the improvement of primary and secondary prevention are required for effective cancer control in LMICs.

   Possible solutions: One way of improving this is to form research collaborative groups involving researchers from LMICs and those from HICs. This will enable the researchers from LMICs to be mentored by researchers from HICs. Such collaborations should focus on identifying common malignancies where obvious improvements can be demonstrated. Senior and junior researchers should be involved in such collaborations, and each team should inculcate research methods, particularly good research practice and good governance, as well as generation of research ideas in LMIC members. There is also the need to improve funding for research to local researchers in LMICs so that they can build their research teams and improve facilities that will enhance research collaborations.

2. Clinical trials provide the main process by which new drugs are introduced into clinical care. There is a need to study individual drugs in target populations to ascertain activity and toxicity in populations because there might be ethnic differences in drug response.

Problem: Less than 2% of global clinical trials in oncology are conducted in sub-Saharan Africa.

In Nigeria, less than five oncology-related clinical trials have been conducted so far based on our search through major clinical trial registration websites. It is also noted that none of the antineoplastic drugs currently in use in Nigeria included indigenous participants in the trial that led to the approval of such agents for use in humans. This implies that the pattern of activity and toxicity of such agents on our population is unknown bearing with it risks for poorer performance and hence poorer acceptance of these drugs.

Solutions: There is a need for collaboration between researchers in HICs with LICs to improve expertise, infrastructure, and support for clinical trials that will involve indigenous populations. All experimentation involving humans must be held to the highest standards, and all principles of good clinical practice must be observed. This is achieved easiest when physicians learn the proper conduct of clinical trials from the best in their fields.

To improve this in Ibadan, we partnered with the University of Chicago, USA, building on a long-standing research collaboration, to improve oncology clinical trials in Nigeria. At the initial survey, there was low capacity of the personnel on the conduct of clinical trials as most of them never took part in a clinical trial before. There were no study monitors conversant with oncology clinical trials to provide regular monitoring of trials to ensure protocol and GCP compliance. There were regulatory bodies in place such as the institutional review boards (IRBs) and the Nigerian national regulatory body—the National Agency for Food and Drug Administration and Control (NAFDAC), but these bodies had limited experience in regulating oncology-related clinical trials. At the institutional levels, there was little experience on the part of the management team on the review and administration of oncology clinical trial contracts. There were also some inadequacies in clinical facilities to support oncology-related trials.

Personnel on all aspects of clinical trial were trained in good clinical practice and relevant areas on Nigerian regulations with respect to clinical trials. The facilitators included personnel from the University of Ibadan, Nigeria, the University of Chicago, and the Roche Pharmaceutical Company. The trained personnel included clinicians, pathologists, radiologists, pharmacists, study coordinators, psycho-oncologists, study nurses, statisticians, data managers, and patient navigators. There were no study monitors and study manager at our center, so six study monitors and one study manager were trained with the assistance of a clinical research organization (CRO) from the USA. During the training, the clinical personnel were able to develop standard operating procedures (SOPs) for their various services. Four centers in Nigeria, which had prior research collaborations with the University of Chicago, were involved in the project. Further details on preparing the sites for clinical trials were captured in our previous report (Ntekim et al. 2020).

To test run our oncology clinical research teams, the University of Chicago sponsored the phase II ARETTA study (ClinicalTrials.gov NCT03879577) to ensure the study teams can deliver. The study is ongoing as at the time of this report under the supervision of the University of Chicago.

There is scarcity of insurance companies in Nigeria with experience in underwriting oncology clinical trials. Therefore, this service was procured in the USA by the University of Chicago. We have, however, identified few indigenous companies in the meantime that have affiliations with US companies capable of providing this service.

Participants' engagement was an issue during the implementation of this trial. Most of the potential participants were not aware of the importance of clinical trials. Enlightenment campaigns were carried out among care groups and nongovernmental organizations to sensitize the populace on clinical trials. This paid off as we were able to enlist the support of these groups thereby improving study accrual.

Infrastructure and Human Resource Development

Infrastructure is crucial in improving oncology care in LMICs.

Problem: There is weak infrastructure for health-care delivery in LMICs including human resource development and retention. Constant overworking leads to a low personnel morale in addition to inadequate supplies of drugs and equipment resulting in brain drain from the subregion.

Possible solution: Part of the efforts by various governments of LMICs must go into upgrading health-care facilities and offering incentives to health-care workers to encourage them to stay. It would be desirable if high-income countries could be assisting by donating up-to-date health-care equipment to support cancer care in LMICs. Training positions can also be made available by high-income countries for oncology health-care personnel from LMICs to have exposure on various aspects of care. Likewise, participation in these pioneering activities might equip personnel from HICs with a unique skillset.

Multidisciplinary Management

Problem: Multidisciplinary management (MDM) is the recommended model for the management of patients with cancer for improved outcome. However, in most LMICs, this model is rarely adopted. This is partly due to inadequate personnel to cover relevant specialties and sometimes due to nonprofessional attitudes. Adoption of precision oncology, which is the current focus for effective cancer management, is currently out of reach in LMICs. This is also related to lack of personnel, infrastructure, and the high cost of targeted therapies that are unaffordable by most patients in LMICs.

Possible solutions: Adoption of multidisciplinary management of patients with cancer should be promoted in LMICs. Where specialists are scarce, mini-tumor boards made up of surgeons, clinical oncologists, pathologists, radiologists, and oncology nurses have been recommended, and virtual attendance should be enabled. This will improve chances of improved review of patients.

This method has been adopted in some centers in Nigeria in the form of site-specific tumor boards. However, few tumor sites, namely, breast, prostate, head, and neck cancers, are covered and even then only in few institutions. There could be linkages with established tumor boards locally and internationally for web-based review of patients to improve clinical management based on established guidelines. Promoting precision medicine in LMICs is possible through establishing partnerships with centers in high-income countries. Samples for molecular analyses could be shipped to centers with facilities and expertise either in-country or in high-income countries for profiling. However, efforts at improving expertise and facilities for precision oncology in LMICs should be pursued passionately. This could start with training on sample preprocessing for shipping to identified labs for analyses.

At present, it would be more feasible and cost-effective to promote early detection thereby enabling local treatment by surgery and/or radiotherapy, first and foremost. This would lead to more in-country competence and nondependence from costly drugs that are currently under scrutiny even in HICs because of their prohibitive cost.

Supportive and Survivorship Care

Palliative care is important in management of patients with cancer, especially in LMICs where most patients present late.

Problem: There is a need to improve pain management and general well-being of the patient as much as possible. These services are hardly available in LMICs.

In Nigeria, for example, palliative care clinics exist in very few centers with none having inpatient care facilities. There are no established training programs on palliative care. Access to pain management and opioid analgesics is still limited.

Possible solution: Training of palliative care experts and provision of palliative care for both inpatients and outpatients must be part of the regular curriculum of human medicine. Efforts should be made to ensure that opioid analgesics are available and affordable to those who need it. Collaboration with relevant institutions is required to upgrade training, infrastructure, and facilities for palliative care services.

There are particular issues associated with survivorship among cancer survivors. Survivors need information concerning their health and social conditions following cancer treatment. The formation of survivor self-help groups has been noted to assist patients greatly toward coping with life after cancer treatment. Such groups are rare in LMICs. Some members of such groups are usually willing to talk about their condition thereby assisting in enlightenment of the populace on cancer and discouraging stigmatization. The formation of survivorship and advocacy groups should be encouraged in LMICs where they can work with health-care personnel and policy makers to promote cancer education and uptake of preventive measures. It is important to change the narrative from one of despair and defeat into one of hope and conquerors.

In Nigeria, the National Cancer Control Plan (2018–2022) contains action plans to address most of the above problems. These include prevention, diagnosis and treatment, hospice/palliative care, and advocacy and mobilization (Federal Ministry of Health 2018). Implementation has, however, fallen short of projections. In the document, the objective was to attain 90% coverage for HPV and HBV vaccination among eligible Nigerians by the year 2022. As at the time of this report, which is about 8 months to the end of year 2022, there is no mass mobilization for HPV and HBV vaccination program in place. Screening of 50% of eligible population for eligible cancer was to be achieved by the year 2022. However, up till now, there has been no change on screening practice in the country. These lapses might relate to inadequate finance, technical capabilities, and perhaps lack of prioritization of cancer services among other economic, sociopolitical, and security challenges in the country.

Conclusion

This chapter described the various challenges associated with the delivery of effective cancer services in LMICs with a focus on Nigeria. Such issues include inadequacies in facilities for prevention, diagnosis, treatment, and follow-up of cancer patients. I highlighted other elements needed for improvement of cancer care such as research and adoption of personalized cancer care and described possible methods of overcoming some of the challenges. These are anchored mainly in collaboration with and support from high-income countries and donor agencies thereby creating also new markets and possibilities of growth within the countries, where these services are being established. Authorities of LMICs also must play important roles in providing infrastructure and formulation of cancer control policies that can be implemented toward improving the outcome of cancer management.

Acknowledgments I wish to acknowledge Ruth und Adolf Merckle Stiftungsfond for supporting my postgraduate training in Advanced Oncology studies at Ulm University, Germany.

References

Barrios CH, Reinert T, Werutsky G (2018) Global breast cancer research: moving forward. Am Soc Clin Oncol Educ Book 38:441–450. https://doi.org/10.1200/edbk_209183

Cazap E et al (2016) Structural barriers to diagnosis and treatment of cancer in low- and middle-income countries: the urgent need for scaling up. J Clin Oncol 34(1):14–19. https://doi.org/10.1200/JCO.2015.61.9189

Delaney G et al (2005) The role of radiotherapy in cancer treatment. Cancer 104(6):1129–1137. https://doi.org/10.1002/cncr.21324

Editors The Lancet Respiratory Medicine (2019) Smoking cessation efforts should target LMICs. Lancet Respir Med 7(9):721. https://doi.org/10.1016/S2213-2600(19)30257-7

El Saghir NS et al (2014) Enhancing cancer care in areas of limited resources: our next steps. Future Oncol 10(12):1953–1965. https://doi.org/10.2217/fon.14.124

Federal Ministry of Health (2018) Nigeria National Cancer Control Plan 2018–2022, Cancer Control

Plan. https://www.iccp-portal.org/system/files/plans/
NCCP_Final%5B1%5D.pdf. Accessed 26 May 2021

Haier J, Sleeman J, Schäfers J (2019) Editorial series:
cancer care in low- and middle-income countries.
Clin Exp Metastasis 36(6):477–480. https://doi.
org/10.1007/s10585-019-10003-4

Hussein WM et al (2016) A review of the infection-
associated cancers in North African countries. Infect
Agents Cancer 11(1):35. https://doi.org/10.1186/
s13027-016-0083-8

IAEA (2020) IAEA and the Global Access to Cancer Care
Foundation to Advance Oncology Training in Low and
Middle Income Countries, Newsletter. https://www.
iaea.org/newscenter/news/iaea-and-the-global-access-
to-cancer-care-foundation-to-advance-oncology-
training-in-low-and-middle-income-countries.
Accessed 26 May 2021

IAEA (2021) Number of Radiotherapy Centers per million people, DIRAC: Directory of Radiotherapy

Centers. https://dirac.iaea.org/Query/Map2?mapId=0.
Accessed 28 May 2021

Katzke VA, Kaaks R, Kühn T (2015) Lifestyle and cancer
risk. Cancer J 21(2):104–110. https://doi.org/10.1097/
PPO.0000000000000101

Ntekim A et al (2020) Implementing oncology clinical
trials in Nigeria: a model for capacity building. BMC
Health Serv Res 20(1):713. https://doi.org/10.1186/
s12913-020-05561-3

Sankaranarayanan R (2014) Screening for cancer ain
low- and middle-income countries. Ann Glob Health
80(5):412. https://doi.org/10.1016/j.aogh.2014.09.014

Shah SC et al (2019) Cancer control in low- and middle-
income countries: is it time to consider screening? J Glob Oncol 5:1–8. https://doi.org/10.1200/
JGO.18.00200

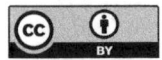

Obstacles and Optimisation of Oncology Services in India

Ninad Katdare

Introduction

The burden of cancer is rapidly increasing in India. India's cancer incidence is estimated at 1.15 million new patients in 2018 and is predicted to almost double as a result of demographic changes alone by 2040. Cancer mortality in India has doubled from 1990 to 2016 (India State-Level Disease Burden Initiative Cancer Collaborators 2018; WHO: Global Cancer Observatory n.d.). It is a crisis of gigantic proportions looming in front of our country. In addition to this, India is the second largest country in terms of population and seventh largest country in terms of size. Additionally, the geography is also varied with very limited access to certain parts of the country like Northeast India. The economic variations are also of gargantuan proportions. Almost 70% of Indians live in small districts and villages, earning not more than 10 dollars per day. Most of it is used for food, clothing and shelter (Devarakonda 2016). In addition to this, the public health spending is abysmal. Only one-fifth of health-care expenditure is publicly financed. The private health sector is a major player; however, insurance awareness as well as

coverage is again dismal, leading to huge out-of-pocket expenses for the patient. Thus, management of cancers in India is a unique scenario with its own challenges. This chapter will cover the various aspects of the obstacles faced and optimisation being carried out at national, local and individual levels.

Historical Perspectives

Cancer in India like in the rest of the world has existed from ancient civilisation. However, no reports were available till the eighteenth century on the prevalence of cancer. The Indian Medical Service staffed by European doctors began to diagnose cancers in the late eighteenth and nineteenth centuries (Crawford 1914). Non-availability or the lack of access to medical facilities where cancer could be diagnosed, cultural habits preventing the use of medical facilities by native Indians, lack of knowledge and skills to diagnose cancer amongst native doctors, lack of compulsory certification of deaths by medical doctors, cover-up of cancer diagnosis because of social stigma and a lack of awareness amongst the native population regarding cancer and its causes and management, also prevented proper registry and data collection (Smith and Mallath 2019). A landmark study across India funded by the Indian Research Fund Association was conducted by Nath et al. in 1939 which showed that cancer was

N. Katdare (✉)
Department of Surgical Oncology, HCG Cancer Centre, Mumbai, Maharashtra, India

U. Schmidt-Strassburger (ed.), *Improving Oncology Worldwide*, Sustainable Development Goals Series, https://doi.org/10.1007/978-3-030-96053-7_14

an important cause of death in all parts of India. This and other factors led to the birth of the Tata Memorial Hospital (TMC) which is considered the apex institute of cancer care in India. It was inaugurated in 1941 (Nath and Grewal KS: Grewal. 1939; Tata Central Archives 1957). Further developments included development of the Cancer Research Institute in 1952 and development of the first population-based cancer registry in 1963. Despite these promising developments in early post-independence India, the manpower and training have fallen woefully short of the exploding population and rapidly increasing number of cancer cases. Whatever workforce is available is heavily skewed towards the private sector and towards urban areas. More than 60% of specialist institutions and specialist are in the southern and western parts of India and in urban India, whereas more than 50% patients of cancer come from the central, eastern and north-eastern regions of India, thus further distorting service provision. From 1990 to present, the cases have doubled, and the death rates have increased by 60% in the same time frame. There is an urgent need to tackle this exploding epidemic.

Cancer Surgery and Surgical Oncology

As a result of the increase in cancer, all public cancer treatment facilities are overcrowded and teeming with patients, resulting in India's cancer problem being called an epidemic. To add to this, there was no central accreditation board for surgical oncology till recently. This led to the development of the so-called part-time cancer surgeon. These were usually general surgeons, ENT (ear, nose and throat) specialists and gynaecologists with a non-formal or limited training in surgical oncology. This lead to substandard and non-standard management of cancer patients. On the other hand, there are also few hundred skilled surgical oncologists at par with one of the best in the world. They are the core "workhorses" who stretch their limits and provide cancer surgeries to cities and towns. However, for the patient population, they are woefully inadequate. This is

compounded by the fact that public health-care spending is meagre coupled with poor infrastructure and the majority of the patients bearing the expenses through out-of-pocket expenditures. This leads to many patients moving to alternative therapies and/or not taking treatment at all.

The Lancet Oncology Commission on Global Cancer Surgery states that over 80% of cancer patients need surgery, some several times (Sullivan et al. 2015). However, providing timely, safe and more importantly affordable surgery is a complex task. It involves health policy decisions, training and management, infrastructure, delivery of care and economic and social issues (Misra et al. 2015). To add to this, there has always been difficulty to do randomised trials in surgery—mostly due to ethical reasons (comparing a surgical versus a sham procedure). Thus, this leads to less than 5% of world's budget being allocated to research in surgical oncology. In developing countries, this is almost non-existent. Till ten years ago, there were very limited training opportunities for surgical oncology in India. This also added to disparities in cancer care delivery.

Obstacles and Optimisation of Oncology Services in India

The mortality: incidence ratio of 0.68 in India is far higher than that in very high human development index (HDI) countries (0.38) and high HDI countries (0.57) (Mallath et al. 2014). The cause for it is manifold. Firstly, there is advanced stage of diagnosis due to illiteracy and lack of awareness; secondly, due to limited access to quality cancer care; and thirdly, the inability of the patient to afford optimum treatment.

Standards of cancer diagnosis and treatment vary considerably between institutions, states and geographical regions. Though regional cancer centres exist in all parts of the country and geographically cover the population, they too have varying standards of care. This lack of uniformity caused patients to travel long distances for optimal care and also caused many patients to leave treatment incomplete due to financial or geographical constraints.

To combat this, various measures are ongoing at various levels—national, local (state) and individual levels.

National: To combat these disparities in standards of care and its availability, the National Cancer Grid (NCG) was formed in August 2012 with the mandate of linking cancer centres across India (Pramesh et al. 2014a). A modest initiative, which originally had 14 cancer centres, has rapidly grown now to include 253 major cancer centres virtually covering the entire length and breadth of the country and is amongst the largest cancer networks in the world. Funded by the Government of India through the Department of Atomic Energy, the NCG has the primary mandate of working towards uniform standards of care across India by adopting evidence-based management guidelines, which are implementable across these centres (Pramesh et al. 2014a).

It has four main objectives (Pramesh et al. 2014a), and these are the following:

1. *Patient care*: To make a set of uniform implementable and simple guidelines for common cancers for easy uptake by the member centres, to make a systematic method of data capture of every patient being treated at a cancer centre and to include a voluntary process of audit and peer review are the steps which will aim to reduce disparities in the standards of patient care in various geographic regions of India.
2. *Education and training:* To create a trained human resource pool, to facilitate exchange of expertise and mentoring between the centres and to have reservation of specialised oncology degree courses for candidates sponsored by the recognised government-run and regional cancer centres, thereby augmenting their trained manpower, are the objectives of education and training.
3. *Collaborative research:* Lack of an established research network was one of the biggest lacunae in cancer care. NCG has already published a comprehensive paper on research priorities in cancer for India (Sullivan et al. 2014) and is working towards that goal.
4. *Cancer policy:* As all the leaders in cancer care, education and research in India are primarily members of the NCG, it is a powerful force to shape cancer policy in India. With the help of its constituent centres, NCG has the natural ability to identify the burden of cancer real time and plan strategies to address specific problems.

Government: To tackle the challenge of non-communicable diseases (NCDs), including cancer, 599 NCD clinics at district level and 3274 NCD clinics at community health centre level have been set up under the National Programme for Prevention and Control of Cancer, Diabetes, Cardiovascular Diseases and Stroke (NPCDCS). Screening of common NCDs including three common cancers, that is, oral, breast and cervical, is also an integral part of service delivery under Ayushman Bharat—Health and Wellness Centres. To enhance the facilities for tertiary care of cancer, the central government is implementing the Strengthening of Tertiary Care for Cancer Scheme, under which setting up of 18 state cancer institutes and 20 tertiary care cancer centres has been approved.

The Tata Memorial Centre through the Department of Atomic Energy (DAE) is setting up six other cancer centres in different parts of the country functioning at par with TMC, Mumbai. These are located in Varanasi (two centres), Guwahati, Sangrur, Vishakhapatnam and Mullanpur. These centres would cater a large number of patients with cancer in all four zones of the country. The two campuses in Mumbai (Parel and Navi Mumbai) are also undergoing expansion in capacity (Anon 2019).

Traditionally, the health-care spending in India was stagnant and just around more than 1% of the GDP. Analysis of the Indian National Health Accounts estimates total health expenditure in India, from all sources, to be about 4.2% of the GDP with 80% being in private sector business (World Bank 2013). However, the health-care allocation has seen a jump of 137% for the fiscal year 2021–2022 as compared to the previous year ushering a small ray of hope. However, planned health investment rarely represents real disbursements, especially when it comes to revenue expenditures in complex disease care such as that for cancer (Mahal et al. 2010).

State: The Indian health-care system is characterised by high rates of privatisation since the 1960s, with low penetration of voluntary and social health insurance schemes and a high frequency of out-of-pocket payments. However, since 2007, the central government and many states in India have started health insurance schemes. These include the Rashtriya Swasthya Bima Yojana (RSBY, a central government initiative), Rajiv Aarogyasri Scheme in Andhra Pradesh, Chief Minister's Comprehensive Health Insurance Scheme in Tamil Nadu, Mahatma Jyotiba Phule Jan Arogya Yojana (MJPJAY) in Maharashtra and Vajpayee Arogyashree Scheme in Karnataka. Though some like the Vajpayee Yojana in Karnataka and Chief Minister's Scheme in Tamil Nadu have met with good success, most of these schemes focus on inpatient care with a low focus on costs from complications and outpatient care. Consequently, out-of-pocket expenses remain high.

Local: Many community-run initiatives such as the Self-Employed Women's Association, Action for Community Organisation, Rehabilitation and Development, Indian Cancer Society and other nongovernmental organisations (NGOs) also support cancer treatment especially for the economically deprived communities. However, many are not designed towards the complexity, costs and delivery of cancer care.

Thus, despite the introduction of government-funded schemes and state and local NGO support, for the average patient with cancer in India, health care remains highly privatised, with more than 80% of outpatient care and 40% of inpatient care provided by the private sector (Pramesh et al. 2014b).

Solutions: Are There Any?

Despite the introduction of government-funded schemes, for the average patient with cancer in India, health care remains highly privatised, with more than 80% of outpatient care and 40% of

inpatient care provided by the private sector (Pramesh et al. 2014b). Roughly 71.7% of health care is financed through out-of-pocket payments (Sullivan et al. 2014; Raghunadharao et al. 2015), with some studies estimating this to be as high as 90% in areas where public health insurance coverage is low (Thakur et al. 2011; Ladusingh and Pandey 2013). Moreover, most out-of-pocket payments are channelled into the private sector, which plays a major part in the provision of health services for outpatient visits (78%) and hospital stays (60%). Consequently, expenditures on private health, especially on drugs, remain very high (Govindarajan and Ramamurti 2013), exacerbating health inequalities. The absence of governance and regulation around private provision of cancer care is creating serious vertical and horizontal imbalances, the classical examples being brain drain to private centres because of attractive salary packages, unnecessary investigations, cherry-picking of patients and non-standardised treatments.

With all these in play, evidence has shown that the high percentage of out-of-pocket payments and low health insurance coverage has resulted in exposure to high financial risk, which pushes patients and their families into catastrophic poverty following a diagnosis of cancer. Almost 50% of patients discontinue treatment because of prohibitive costs. Around 10% of rural households become poorer because of out-of-pocket cancer costs.

So how do we combat this "epidemic"? In the public sector, the National Cancer Grid is taking phenomenal strides to achieve an equitable distribution of cancer care. There are few public-private (philanthropic) initiatives also in play. The private sector can also contribute in various ways. Only then can the entire scenario for cancer care change in India.

The following steps can go a long way in improving the cancer care in India:

National Cancer Grid (NCG) Initiatives

The following initiatives have already been started by the NCG to combat the problems in the delivery of cancer care (Pramesh et al. 2014a; Sullivan et al. 2014; Pramesh et al. 2014b; Pramesh et al. 2019; Raghunadharao et al. 2015):

(a) Adoption of implementable resource stratified guidelines.
(b) Systematic method of data capture at all centres as part of the grid.
(c) A voluntary process of audit and peer review: This is a unique initiative by the NCG as, in India, accreditation and peer review in Indian health-care providers have been the exception rather than the rule. Though accreditations like JCI (Joint Commission International) and NABH (National Accreditation Board for Hospitals) exist in India, they are mainly focused towards processes, systems and documentation rather than the medical aspect of health care. Few centres have already completed the review, and few centres are in the process of getting the review done. This will go a long way in standardisation of cancer care in India.
(d) Exchange of expertise and mentoring between member centres of NCG.
(e) Plan varying durations of training for physicians and paramedical staff to augment human resource.
(f) To increase number of training opportunities for specialist and to have reservation for government-run and regional cancer centres to augment their trained manpower.
(g) To prioritise research topics in Indian context and development of established research networks.
(h) To formulate a national cancer plan to improve the mortality: incidence ratio.
(i) Choosing Wisely India: The Choosing Wisely India is an initiative modelled after the Choosing Wisely in the USA and Canada but tailored to the Indian context (Pramesh et al. 2019). It has identified ten low-value and potentially harmful practices in the Indian cancer care scenario. The recommendations have been endorsed by all major cancer centres in India and the NCG.

Public Sector: Philanthropic Initiatives

Tata Trusts—one of India's oldest, non-sectarian philanthropic organisations—is working in partnership with multiple state governments and central government to roll out a step-down, distributed cancer care model. The first state to reach implementation stage is Assam—a state in Northeast India, where the programme is jointly funded by the government of Assam and Tata Trusts. In this model, smaller centres interlinked with the apex centres through a technology backbone will handle diagnosis and care delivery (Anon n.d.-a; Anon n.d.-b).

Though cancer drug pricing is low in India, after calculating prices as a percentage of wealth adjusted for the cost of living, cancer drugs appeared to be least affordable in India and China. Also a market analysis recently revealed that there are many interhospital variations and peculiarities in the pricing of cancer drugs. This has promoted the setting up of a "Price Discovery Cell" which is a joint initiative of the Tata Trusts and NCG. The aim is to promote informed buying by the hospitals and also to consolidate buying by pooling demand and having economies of scale (Anon n.d.-b).

Private Sector Initiatives

The last decade has seen an explosion in the developments in the fields of medical, surgical and radiation oncology. Developments like immunotherapy, robotic therapy and proton therapy though latest do not always translate into best results and benefits to patients. In most emerging economies, there is a chronic underuse of therapies that can save lives (such as cervical cancer screening, basic surgery and radiotherapy) and a chronic overuse of interventions that, at huge expense to the patient, provide no meaningful benefit. This leads to inflated health-care costs in the private sector. Add to this the discrepancy in cancer drug pricing which takes the costs of cancer care in private sector through the roof. However, a change in the mindset and few changes in the way health care is delivered in private sector can make health care affordable, available and also profitable. This in the long run can also improve private sector participation in tackling the "epidemic" of cancer. The following techniques can go a long way in reducing the cost of cancer care in private sector which in turn can also reduce the burden on the public sector hospitals (Mir 2017; Anon n.d.-c).

(a) *Focused processes and performance management*: This includes not only standardisation of operational processes but also clinical processes. With involvement of the clinician in standardisation of clinical process, the outcomes improve, and morbidity goes down. This in turn helps in improved throughput of operating rooms and operational beds thus getting down the costs. The use of information technology and analytics can further help refining the process and delivering more robust performance.

(b) *Integrated processes*: Most organisations look at capital allocation and returns separately, with limited accountability through processes such as performance look-backs that track value created as compared to only cost of capital. Improved capital allocation should be strategically integrated with operational execution, measuring financial return over time to identify the need for process improvement and/or other strategic levels. The agility to boost return on underperforming clinical assets by applying smart strategies is a capability that will drive increasing value and at the same time help keep costs down paving way for affordable health care.

(c) *Promoting innovations that suit local conditions*: With the "Make in India" initiative promoted by the government, many devices and drugs are being now made in India at fraction of the cost required for importing those. The use of such "indigenous" capital intensive items can reduce the initial capital allocation and requirement thus promoting earlier return on investment (ROI) even while keeping the cost of treatment low. The classical examples in cancer care being the use of indigenous retractors, indigenous "HIPEC" (hyperthermic intraperitoneal chemotherapy) machines and indigenous chemotherapy ports.

(d) *Investment in human resource rather than material resource*: At higher centres, highly skilled doctors and paramedical staff are trained to do more skilled work. This improves clinical outcome and also improves efficiency, thus increasing the throughput. At the other end of the spectrum, training non-skilled or semi-skilled workers to take on paramedical responsibilities can help in outreach services and also provide basic care to the remote parts of the country.

(e) *Patient empowerment*: This includes empowering patients and their caretakers to take a more active role in managing their conditions, while enabling greater differentiation of services based on needs and desired outcomes. For example, head and neck cancer patients and relatives are taught with tube feeding and oral care which enables self-sufficiency at an earlier stage. This combined with home care by a trained home care team helps in reducing the patient's hospital stay and costs and at the same time increasing the turnover of beds leading to both affordable and profitable care.

(f) *Building scale:* Increasing operating scale helps health-care providers in several ways: it supports the expansion of services, leads to improved asset and staff utilisation and enables increased investment in IT, performance management and new ways of working.

(g) *Asserting frugality*: This has been traditionally being done in Indian hospitals, where a single-use device is sterilised and used multiple times. As long as strict sterilisation norms are being followed, studies have shown that there has been no increase in morbidity or complications (Sullivan et al. 2017). This however often gets used to build up the ROI. However, if these get utilised towards reducing treatment costs, then more affordable cancer care can be delivered.

Hub and Spoke Model

For a country like the size of India, with its geographical, demographic and social variations, the only way to have uniform and accessible cancer care delivery is by the hub and spoke model. This coupled with the use of information technology, and social media can go a long way in not only delivery of care but also in spreading awareness and preventive measures (Devarakonda 2016).

On the backbone of the NCG, the private sector hospitals can also have a hub and spoke model. With the advent of many cancer treatment-specific hospitals, with proper use of resources and the points outlined in the previous section, an attempt can be made to make health care more affordable in private sector. The NCG can be a governing body for all the cancer hospitals in private sector to ensure uniformity of care. The "hubs" can be established in all major metropolitan cities with certain megacities and megalopolis like Mumbai and Delhi-NCR having more than one hub. These centres should invest in all latest technologies which may prove to be cost-effective if they get feeders from all their spokes. Moreover, there will be a focused group of dedicated specialists available here which can translate into improved outcomes for complex as well as esoteric cases.

The biggest advantage for cancer care is that because of the highly specialised nature of the treatment plans and protocols, it lends itself to formation of highly itemised standard operating procedures (SOPs). The use of these SOPs can make the management of standard and early cancers easier to learn and adopt even for non-formally trained doctors like general surgeons, gynaecologists, etc. With the help of NCG and the various "hubs," these doctors can be trained to manage patients in the tier 1 and tier 2 "spokes." In the most remote corners, non-allopathy doctors and paramedical staff can be trained to detect cancer at an early stage and refer to the tier 1 and tier 2 "spokes" (Devarakonda 2016).

It has also been seen that in India, a big factor adding to the cost of drugs and consumables is the fragmented and inefficient supply chain. As a percentage of cost of goods sold, the average sup-ply chain cost of the pharmaceutical industry in India is 25% as compared to 10% globally. Supply chain efficiencies and tie-ups with the entire hub and spoke model can create economies of scale which will also bring cost of drugs down. This coupled with the "Price Cell" initiative of NCG can help drive the costs down further (Anon n.d.-b).

A recent update from the Telecom authorities of India showed that there are almost 1175 million mobile users as of December 2020 with over 800 million users having Internet connectivity (Telecom Regulatory Authority of India 2021). The advent of COVID-19 has expanded the reach of telemedicine. The use of this information technology can be used not only to spread awareness but also provide training to non-allopathy medical practitioners and paramedical staff. It can also be used to transfer encrypted patient's data between the "hubs," "spokes" and grassroot-level staff for second-opinion and treatment planning where trained staff is not available. This can thus ensure delivery of quality cancer care to the most remote parts of India too.

Certain hospital networks like the Narayana Hrudayalaya for cardiac care and Aravind Eye Hospitals for eye care have shown that such models work even in the private sector and can make health care affordable as well as profitable at the same time ensuring reach to the more remote parts of India (Govindarajan and Ramamurti 2013).

Conclusion

The misuse of technology in cancer care for profit is a major issue in many countries where health care is unregulated (Pramesh et al. 2014b). Developing country-specific management guidelines and linking government insurance reimbursements to adherence to these could further encourage providers to deliver evidence-based care (Sullivan et al. 2017). This work has been started in a great way by the NCG. Systems of accreditation for cancer centres both in the public and private domains could also help to ensure that institutions offer interventions only after demonstrating competence and achieving certain scores from patient's feedback and peer review. Combining these policies in a hub and spoke model coupled with the use of information technology can definitely help in expanding the reach while minimising costs.

Involving the private sector and connecting private capital to a market orientation can bring efficiency to health-care provision while delivering high-quality, affordable health care to those in need. This has been well exemplified in the aviation sector wherein low-cost models have boosted the development of business models which are more profitable than their conventional peers. The use of techniques mentioned above can make cancer care available, affordable and even profitable (in the private sector) thus augmenting the reach and efforts of the public sector.

The director of Tata Memorial Hospital, the oldest and largest cancer hospital in India, has rightly said.

"Cancer 'Moonshots' may improve individual outcomes in developed countries , but what India needs is Cancer "Earthshots" that are focused on building infrastructure and delivering effective, evidence based, equitable and more importantly affordable cancer care" (Sullivan et al. 2017).

References

Anon (2019). https://pib.gov.in/Pressreleaseshare.aspx?PRID=1596310. Accessed 26 Jan 2021

Anon (n.d.-a). https://horizons.tatatrusts.org/2019/march/cancer-care-distributed-care-model.html. Accessed 20 Feb 2021

Anon (n.d.-b). https://www.devex.com/news/opinion-a-new-model-of-distributed-accessible-affordable-cancer-care-in-india-93376. Accessed 20 Feb 2021

Anon (n.d.-c) ge-healthcare-white paper -boosting returns.pdf. Accessed 12 Mar 2021

Crawford DG (1914) A history of the Indian medical service, 1600–1913. London, Thacker. https://archive.org/details/b21352148/page/n15/mode/2up. Accessed 18 Jan 2021

Devarakonda S (2016) Hub and spoke model: making rural health care in India affordable, available and accessible. Rural Remote Health 16(1):3476. Epub 2016 Feb 3

Govindarajan V, Ramamurti R (2013) Delivering world-class health care, afford-ably. Harv Bus Rev 2. http://hbr.org/2013/11/delivering-world-class-health-care-affordably/ar/1

India State-Level Disease Burden Initiative Cancer Collaborators (2018) The burden of cancers and their variations across the states of India: the Global Burden of Disease Study 1990–2016. Lancet Oncol 19(10):1289–1306. https://doi.org/10.1016/S1470-2045(18)30447-9. Epub 2018 Sep 12. Erratum in: Lancet Oncol. 2018;: PMID: 30219626; PMCID: PMC6167407

Ladusingh L, Pandey A (2013) Health expenditure and impoverishment in India. J Health Manag 15(1):57–74. https://doi.org/10.1177/0972063413486031

Mahal A, Karan A, Engelgau M (2010) The Economic Implications of Non-Communicable Disease for India. Health, Nutrition and Population (HNP) discussion paper;. World Bank, Washington, DC. © World Bank. https://openknowledge.worldbank.org/handle/10986/13649. License: CC BY 3.0 IGO

Mallath MK, Taylor DG, Badwe RA, Rath GK, Shanta V, Pramesh CS et al (2014) The growing burden of cancer in India: epidemiology and social context. Lancet Oncol 15:e205–e212. https://doi.org/10.1016/S1470-2045(14)70115-9. Epub 2014 Apr 11

Mir A (2017) Making affordable healthcare profitable. Health management.org. Journal 17(2)

Misra S, Agarwal A, Chaturvedi A (2015) Cancer surgery: an Indian-Asian perspective. Lancet Oncol 16(11):1189–1190. https://doi.org/10.1016/S1470-2045(15)00277-6

Nath V, Grewal KS: Grewal. (1939) Cancer in India. Indian J Med Res 26:785–832

Pramesh CS, Badwe RA, Sinha RK (2014a) The national cancer grid of India. Indian J Med Paediatr Oncol 35(3):226–227. https://doi.org/10.4103/0971-5851.142040. PMID: 25336795; PMCID: PMC4202620

Pramesh CS, Badwe RA, Borthakur BB, Chandra M, Raj EH, Kannan T et al (2014b) Delivery of affordable and equitable cancer care in India. Lancet Oncol 15:e223–e233. https://doi.org/10.1016/S1470-2045(14)70117-2. Epub 2014 Apr 11

Pramesh CS, Chaturvedi H, Reddy VA, Saikia T, Ghoshal S, Pandit M et al (2019) National cancer grid. Choosing Wisely India: ten low-value or harmful practices that should be avoided in cancer care. Lancet Oncol 20(4):e218–e223. https://doi.org/10.1016/S1470-2045(19)30092-0. Epub 2019 Mar 8

Raghunadharao D, Kannan R, Hingnekar C, Vijaykumar DK, Mani CS, Ghosh-Laskar S, National Cancer Grid et al (2015) Institutional external peer review: a unique National Cancer Grid initiative. Indian J Med Paediatr Oncol 36(3):186–188. https://doi.org/10.4103/0971-5851.166753. PMID: 26855528; PMCID: PMC4743180

Smith RD, Mallath MK (2019) History of the growing burden of cancer in India: from antiquity to the 21st century. J Glob Oncol 5:1–15. https://doi.org/10.1200/JGO.19.00048. PMID: 31373840; PMCID: PMC7010436

Sullivan R, Badwe RA, Rath GK, Pramesh CS, Shanta V, Digumarti R et al (2014) Cancer research in India: national priorities, global results. Lancet Oncol 15(6):e213–e222. https://doi.org/10.1016/S1470-2045(14)70109-3. Epub 2014 Apr 11

Sullivan R, Alatise OI, Anderson BO, Audisio R, Autier P, Aggarwal A et al (2015) Global cancer surgery: delivering safe, affordable, and timely cancer surgery. Lancet Oncol 16(11):1193–1224. https://doi.org/10.1016/S1470-2045(15)00223-5

Sullivan R, Pramesh CS, Booth CM (2017) Cancer patients need better care, not just more technology. Nature 549(7672):325–328. https://doi.org/10.1038/549325a

Tata Central Archives (1957) Box 181, Appendix A Tata Memorial Hospital. Pune, India, Tata Central. http://www.tatacentralarchives.com/. Accessed 18 Jan 2021

Telecom Regulatory Authority of India (2021) Highlights of Telecom Subscription Data; 1. https://www.trai.gov.in/sites/default/files/PR_No.06of2021_0.pdf. Accessed 12 Mar 2021

Thakur J, Prinja S, Garg CC, Mendis S, Menabde N (2011) Social and economic implications of noncommunicable diseases in India. Indian J Community Med 36(Suppl 1):S13–S22. https://doi.org/10.4103/0970-0218.94704. PMID: 22628905; PMCID: PMC3354895

WHO: Global Cancer Observatory (n.d.) International Agency for Research on Cancer. https://gco.iarc.fr/. Accessed 10 Jan 2021

World Bank (2013) World development indicators. http://data.worldbank.org/indicator/SH.XPD.PUBL. Accessed 26 Jan 2021

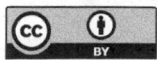

Integrating Palliative Care into Primary Care: An Educational Project to Meet an Unmet Need

Amir Radfar

Background and Significance

Palliative care is considered one of the pillars of cancer control and plays an essential role in managing cancer complications and treatment. Per the World Health Organization (WHO), palliative care is defined as a series of measures to improve the quality of life of patients and their families and to solve problems associated with the incurable life-threatening illness through the prevention or relief of suffering employing an early diagnosis and the assessment and treatment of pain and other psychological, physical, and spiritual problems (World Health Organization (WHO) 2021). Palliative care and pain relief are considered essential elements of universal health coverage (UHC).

Primary Palliative Care Versus Subspecialty Palliative Care

Palliative care can be offered by palliative care specialists who work alongside the patients' primary care physician and is known as subspecialty palliative care, which is now recognized as a med-ical subspecialty in many countries. The specialty of palliative care is mostly available in high-income countries but is generally quite limited in the middle- and low-income countries (Poudel et al. 2019). Alternatively, clinicians who are not palliative care specialists can offer palliative care for seriously ill patients and provide basic palliative care. These palliative care services are called primary or basic palliative care. They may include basic pain management, basic management of other physical symptoms, basic use of adjuvant pain relievers, basic care coordination, and seriously ill patients' routine care. Primary palliative care can foster clinician-patient relationships, reduce care fragmentation, alleviate pain and suffering, and provide empathic care (Quill and Abernethy 2013). However, primary care physicians require basic palliative care competencies and skills to provide disease management and symptom palliation (Bowman and Meier 2018).

Palliative Care in Iran: Past, Present, and Future

Iran, with a population of 82.8 million, among which 70% are aged 15–64 and 6% are aged 65 or older, is located in Western Asia (Fig. 1) (World Bank 2021a, b, c, d; Plecher 2021). Cancer is the third leading cause of death in Iran, and given the increasing life expectancy, the WHO estimated a cancer mortality of 62,000 in

A. Radfar (✉)
Medical Education, University of Central Florida, Orlando, FL, USA
e-mail: aradf001@fiu.edu

U. Schmidt-Strassburger (ed.), *Improving Oncology Worldwide*, Sustainable Development Goals Series,
https://doi.org/10.1007/978-3-030-96053-7_15

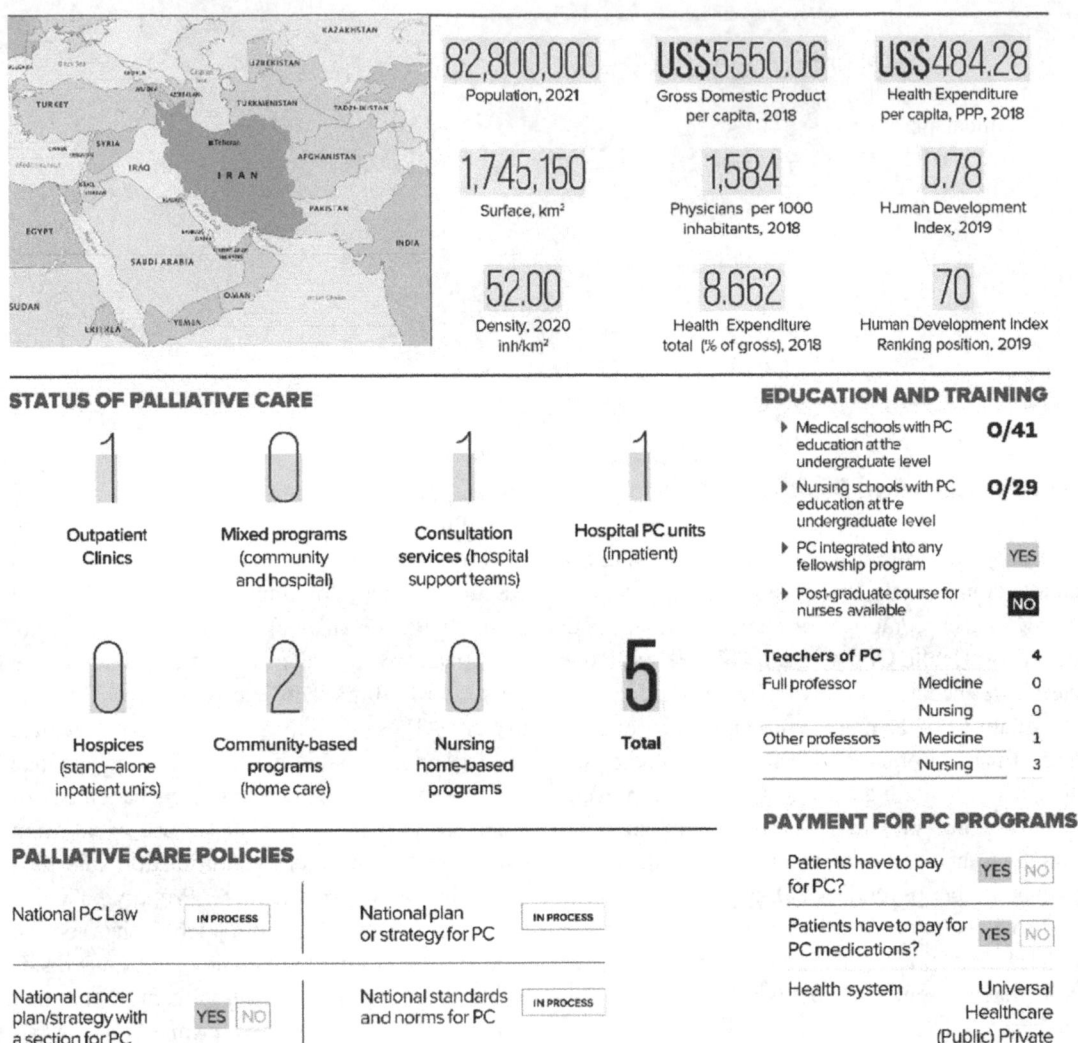

Fig. 1 Demographics and status of palliative care services and training in Iran (World Bank 2021a; World Bank 2021b; World Bank 2021c; World Bank 2021d; United Nations Development Program (UNDP) 2019; Osman et al. 2017). (Persiannfin.com. Persian in Finland. (2022). Retrieved from http://persianfinn.com/persian-speaking-in-finland/)

the year 2020. Currently, 300,000 cancer patients live, and 109,000 individuals have added to this number annually (Keyghobadi et al. 2015). The northern part of the country is a known area with a high incidence of gastric and esophageal cancer (Ghasemi et al. 2020).

The history of palliative care in Iran dates back to the 1920s, when the first hospice for leprosy patients was established (Mojen 2017). However, modern palliative care for cancer dates back to the year 2000, when trained palliative care experts collaborated with the Royal Hospital for Women in Australia and led a series of workshops and trained specialists in palliative medicine with the Sydney Institute of Palliative Medicine (Mojen 2017). Counseling services for palliative care were established in the Cancer Research Center in Tehran in 2006 and other provincial services in different provinces in the subsequent years (Mojen 2017). These services offer subspecialized palliative care at the tertiary level to the public (Fig. 1). Several charity organizations also provide palliative care to both patients and their families and are mostly run by volunteers (Mojen 2017).

Integrating palliative subspecialty training into clinical practice was established through a palliative medicine fellowship program in 2012 and is up and running as of now. One to two palliative care specialists graduate each year (Fig. 1).

Medical universities are increasingly adopting a palliative medicine curriculum for the medical residents, and palliative care subjects also became a required component of any oncology conference in the country. However, palliative care services do not follow a systematic structure, and primary palliative care in Iran is in its infancy. The lack of an organized system to provide palliative care services is partly due to a shortage of trained primary care providers such as general practitioners and nurses who are the backbone of a well-established public health network.

With the increased number of the elderly population, providing palliative care for other age-related diseases such as advanced heart failure, advanced pulmonary disease, and dementia is an ongoing challenge for the public health system. Shortages of pediatrics primary palliative care services and partial coverage of these services by insurance companies make the issue even more complicated.

Primary Palliative Care Educational Project

The development of the evidence-based, culturally sensitive primary palliative care content material in Farsi (the language spoken in Iran and some other Central Asian countries) for general practitioners is the main objective of an ongoing educational pilot project. Knowledge obtained from the training in the advanced oncology program at the University of Ulm, Germany, in addition to collaboration with the Center for Palliative Medicine at the University Hospital of Cologne, Germany, is the principal motive behind an initiative to create an online educational platform in Farsi for 30 primary care providers.

The educational content would be provided for the volunteer physicians working in cancer care and includes palliative care subject matter. This pilot study's educational contents are being verified by subject matter experts addressing the current challenges in primary palliative care. These educational subjects include the physical, psychological, social, and spiritual sources of pain and suffering experienced by patients and their families. Modules on pain and symptom management, interdisciplinary teamwork and collaboration among disciplines, communication skills, special needs of patients at various stages of the life cycle, bereavement, practices toward the end of life, and ethical and legal subjects will be soon made available to the general practitioners. The educational materials will be updated continuously on an online platform, and a certificate of attendance will be offered to the participants. This pilot project could eventually be extended as a model for establishing an educational platform of primary palliative care for other Farsi-speaking populations worldwide.

This project distinguishes itself through the following characteristics:

- Specific: It is a pilot study to design a culturally sensitive educational content material in palliative care for volunteer general practitioners in Farsi.
- Measurable: A posttest-only assessment of acquired knowledge would be performed through an online medium.
- Attainable: The content would be adapted from the international evidence-based practices and guidelines. However, based on local expertise and knowledge, it will highlight the role of cultural competence.
- Relevant: The content material would be used for continuous medical education in primary palliative care in Farsi.
- Time: This one-year pilot project was planned to be started in 2019, but due to an unforeseen severe COVID-19 pandemic, it was postponed, continuing in 2022.

Challenges

Besides the COVID-19 pandemic's logistic limitations, this project anticipates further challenges such as the inability to secure funding and reliance on volunteerism, bureaucratic procedures, and the existence of competing palliative and pain management subspecialty programs, which do not share the same concept as the primary palliative care. The lack of confidence in completing the participants' educational tasks and the time pressure are additional hindering factors to be considered (Barclay et al. 2019).

Conclusion

Although significant steps have been taken toward comprehensive palliative care in Farsi speaking countries such as Iran, there is a big gap between the status quo and the optimal state. Palliative care for patients with cancer is a significant challenge faced by the patients, their families, and healthcare providers. Given the increased life expectancy and aging of the population, cancer incidence is expected to double over the next two decades. The increased mortality and morbidity rates for patients with cancer, proven efficacy, and better clinical outcomes demand comprehensive palliative care services. Improving the health and quality of life in these patients and their families makes primary palliative care necessary.

The prospect of the primary palliative care in Farsi speaking countries relies on education and training for the primary care providers, developing a standard of the care service package and an independent discipline of primary palliative and supportive care. The establishment of evidence-based, culturally sensitive primary palliative care educational material in Farsi can address shortages of the trained workforce in primary palliative care. Research in palliative care to provide a regional palliative care model based on domestic resources and availabilities is pivotal for optimal survivorship and palliative care. As part of the curriculum for medical, nursing, and other relevant disciplines, primary palliative care training and creating an international link for training and research to develop palliative care services are among other venues to pursue.

Acknowledgments We thank Doctor Uta Schmidt-Straßburger, a scientific director of the Advanced Oncology Program at Ulm University, Germany, for her continuous support; the University of Ulm, Germany, for fostering continuous postgraduate learning in oncology; Doctor Irina Filip, an assistant professor of Clinical Psychiatry at Western University of Medical Sciences, Pomona, USA and Doctor Mamak Tahmasebi, an attending physician and palliative care specialist, Tehran, Iran, for their meaningful comments; and the European Palliative Care Academy and the Ruth and Adolf Merckle Foundation and DAAD (German Academic Exchange Service), Germany, for their generous educational support.

References

Barclay S, Moran E, Boase S, Johnson M, Lovick R, Graffy J, White PL, Deboys B, Harrison K, Swash B (2019) Primary palliative care research: opportunities and challenges. BMJ Support Palliat Care 9(4):468–472

Bowman B, Meier DE (2018) Palliative care for respiratory disease: an education model of care. Chron Respir Dis 15(1):36–40

Ghasemi S, Dreassi E, Aghamohammadi S, Mahaki B (2020) Mapping spatial variation of the stomach, esophageal and lung cancers and their shared risk factors in Iran at a county level. https://doi.org/10.21203/rs.3.rs-59536/v1

Keyghobadi N, Rafiemanesh H, Mohammadian-Hafshejani A, Enayatrad M, Salehiniya H (2015) Epidemiology and trend of cancers in the province of Kerman: southeast of Iran. Asian Pac J Cancer Prev 16(4):1409–1413

Mojen LK (2017) Palliative care in Iran: the past, the present and the future. Support PalliatCare Cancer 1(1)

Osman H, Rihan A, Garralda E, Rhee JY, Pons-Izquierdo JJ, Lima L, Tfayli A, Centeno C (2017) Atlas of palliative care in the Eastern Mediterranean region. https://dadun.unav.edu/handle/10171/43303. Accessed 28 Feb 2021

Plecher H (2021) Age structure in Iran 2009–2019. https://www.statista.com/statistics/294213/iran-age-structure/#:~:text=This%20statistic%20shows%20the%20age,were%20aged%2065%20or%20older. Accessed 28 Feb 2021

Poudel A, Bhuvan KC, Shrestha S, Nissen L (2019) Access to palliative care: discrepancy among low-income and high-income countries. J Glob Health 9(2):020309

Quill TE, Abernethy AP (2013) Generalist plus specialist palliative care—creating a more sustainable model. N Engl J Med 368(13):1173–1175

United Nations Development Program (UNDP) (2019) Human development report 2019: beyond income, beyond averages, beyond today. https://www.ir.undp.org/content/iran/en/home/presscenter/articles/2019/Human-Development-Report-2019.html. Accessed 28 Feb 2021

World Bank (2021a) Iran overview. https://www.worldbank.org/en/country/iran/overview. Accessed 28 Feb 2021

World Bank (2021b) Physician Iran data. https://data.worldbank.org/. Accessed 28 Feb 2021

World Bank (2021c) Population density. https://data.worldbank.org/. Accessed 28 Feb 2021

World Bank (2021d) Current health expenditure Iran https://data.worldbank.org/. Accessed 28 Feb 2021

World Health Organization (WHO) (2021) Palliative care. https://www.who.int/health-topics/palliative-care. Accessed 28 Feb 2021

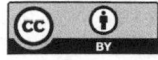

Challenges in Developing Pediatric Cancer Care in Armenia

Gevorg Tamamyan

Parallel Worlds

When I was born, pediatric cancer was considered incurable in Armenia. It was 1987.

In the same year, Steinherz from Cornell wrote in his manuscript that "over the last 20 years, the rate of long-term disease-free survival of childhood acute lymphoblastic leukemia increased from less than 1 to 60 per cent" (Steinherz 1987).

When I entered medical school in 2004, the survival rate of pediatric acute lymphoblastic leukemia (ALL) in Armenia was already close to 65% (Danielyan 2009; Danielyan and Iskanyan 2004). At that very moment, I even did not know what leukemia is; that word was familiar to me only from a South American soap opera, and in my memory, it was associated with a beautiful girl, who was bald and sometimes sad.

According to the World Health Organization (WHO), in the high-income countries (HIC), the survival rate of pediatric cancer is around 80%, meaning that four out of five children with cancer survive. However, in the low- and middle-income countries (LMIC), the situation is opposite, meaning that four out of five children with cancer die (Childhood Cancer n.d.).

On February 15, 2021, on the International Childhood Cancer Day, I gave an interview and reported a survival rate of pediatric cancer in Armenia close to 75% (Tamamyan 2020; Hovhannisyan et al. 2020; Papyan 2018). To me it was an achievement, achievement of hard work and dedication of a beautiful team of doctors and nurses, who made this happen. Armenia, a developing country with very limited resources, is reporting pediatric cancer survival close to the HIC. Currently, I am fortunate to lead the only institution in Armenia treating children with hematologic and oncologic disorders; that wonderful team made this miracle happen. But 17 years ago, at that very moment, I even could not imagine that one day, in one of the early Armenian mornings, I would be sitting in the office of the Pediatric Cancer and Blood Disorders Center of Armenia and writing this chapter about the challenges and achievements of pediatric cancer care in Armenia.

In this chapter, I will try to present the work of the generations of pediatric hematologists and oncologists, who made the treatment of pediatric cancer care in Armenia a reality, about the challenges and hardships and about the achievements and future plans.

G. Tamamyan (✉)
Pediatric Cancer and Blood Disorders Center of Armenia, Hematology Center After Prof. R.H. Yeolyan, Yerevan, Armenia

Department of Pediatric Oncology and Hematology, Yerevan State Medical University, Yerevan, Armenia

Master Program in Advanced Oncology, University of Ulm, Ulm, Germany

© The Author(s) 2022
U. Schmidt-Strassburger (ed.), *Improving Oncology Worldwide*, Sustainable Development Goals Series, https://doi.org/10.1007/978-3-030-96053-7_16

From 0.7% to 80%

Armenia is a small country in South Caucasus, with a population of three million. For several thousand years, starting back from Noah, Armenians have been living on this land and throughout the whole history of humanity experienced many rises and falls. The current Republic of Armenia declared its independence in 1991, after the collapse of the Soviet Union (Wikipedia: Armenia n.d.). The devastating earthquake of 1988, which destroyed the whole northern part of the country and killed more than 38,000 people, the Nagorno–Karabakh war, thousands of refugees, closed borders, and collapsed post-Soviet economy contributed to the situation when in 1992–1994, several pediatric hematologists at the Hematology Center named after Prof. R.H. Yeolyan (previously called Scientific Research Institute of Hematology and Blood Transfusion) started thinking about doing multiagent chemotherapy for children with leukemias.

Dr. Samvel Danielyan, a newly appointed chief of the pediatric hematology department, returned from Moscow and, together with the medical and nursing team of the department, started the German BFM treatment protocol for children with ALL. Lack of cancer medications, supportive care agents, and infusion pumps and limited electricity, water, and blood supply are the contributing factors which were guarantees for the failure. But, as it was well said, where there is a will, there is a way, and children started getting into remission and more and more started getting cured.

Recently, it was published that from 1982 till 1994, only 3 (0.7%) out of 430 children with ALL in Armenia survived, but after the implementation of BFM protocol, between 1994 and 2019 years, 502 (73.3%) out of 685 children with ALL conquered leukemia (Danielyan et al. 2020). The results were impressive and comparable with the results from the Western developed countries.

Therapeutic treatment of patients with pediatric solid tumors was organized at the National Oncology Center, as well as the radiation therapy department that was located there. Surgeries were performed in several public and private pediatric hospitals.

In 2008, part of the team led by Dr. Danielyan, involving also young physicians just after completing fellowship training, moved to the Muratsan Hospital of Yerevan State Medical University, where not only children with hematologic malignancies but also children with solid tumors started getting treatment according to the internationally recognized treatment schemes. This, in turn, led to better outcomes in this group of patients. A recent analysis from Muratsan Hospital showed a 5-year overall survival close to 80% (Tamamyan 2020; Papyan 2018).

Entering a New World

In September 2010, I walked the doors of the Clinic of Chemotherapy of Muratsan Hospital of YSMU as a first year fellow of hematology. At that time, we did not have a separate fellowship program for pediatric hematology–oncology. So, to treat children with cancer, you had to finish either the hematology (3 years) or oncology (2 years) fellowship program, which included both adult and pediatric parts. Childhood leukemias were the most interesting for me, so I chose the hematology fellowship, but doing it at the oncology department led by Dr. Danielyan.

The clinic was on the first floor of a pediatric academic hospital on the edge of Yerevan City. It was handed over to the university several years ago and had been actively in the reorganization and construction processes. The chemotherapy clinic had both pediatric and adult practices, so physicians were treating children and adults with different malignancies. Opinions were different about a joint pediatric and adult clinic. Some were saying it was a bad idea to have them together; others were saying the opposite, especially after seeing happy faces of adult patients after the interaction with their new little friends. But I can surely say, at that very moment, it was a very productive cooperation and led to major changes in the cancer care in Armenia.

During my student years, I had classes in majority of the hospitals in Armenia, but the Muratsan Hospital and the Clinic of Chemotherapy were something different. The atmosphere, the team, and the dedicated people—all these were making this place unique. In Armenia—and I am sure in many other developing countries—cancer is stigmatized, and the majority of people associate it with a death sentence. People visit cancer centers very depressed and sad, but one thing I clearly remember from Muratsan is that people were telling that this clinic is different that you get so much positive energy there.

This positive energy caught me as well, and from the first moment I entered the clinic, I became part of Muratsan and part of that exceptional team.

Getting Around the Globe

Besides being a team, where every member was helping each other, the Muratsan team also was very active on getting training outside of Armenia. Dr. Danielyan had always been telling that we needed to see the world and to observe and learn how people practice medicine in the other countries—this would be the only way to become a good specialist and to improve our field of medicine in our country. Not surprisingly, it was not a common practice in Armenia, and I think in many other developing countries, to encourage your team members to get around the world and invest in education. Usually it is opposite; supervisors try to oppress the youngsters, thereby often eliminating the future competition.

When people ask me "What is the key for your success?" I would always say without any hesitation that I was fortunate to have the best mentors one could imagine, and this was true starting from Armenia going to the USA, Germany, Taiwan, Austria, and Belgium.

During the recent 10 years, I do not remember a single day, when I was not a student. Currently, I am leading a pediatric cancer center, chairing a department at the medical university, and just recently got a full professorship, but right now also, I am a student, studying global health diplomacy at Toronto University (Canada).

For me education has never been just merely a knowledge gaining process but also a way of exploring the world, becoming acquainted with people, interacting with them and using the knowledge and skills, and, most importantly, networking to improve the cancer care in my country.

It has been a long journey for me—visiting fellowships in pediatric hematology/oncology at the Children's Hospital of China Medical University (Taichung, Taiwan), St. Anna Children's Hospital (Vienna, Austria), master's program in advanced oncology at the University of Ulm (Ulm, Germany), PhD fellowship in oncology at YSMU (Yerevan, Armenia), postdoctoral fellowship in the leukemia department at the University of Texas MD Anderson Cancer Center (Houston, TX, USA), medical research fellowship at the European Organization for Research and Treatment of Cancer Headquarters (Brussels, Belgium), visiting scientist at the Dana–Farber/Boston Children's Cancer and Blood Disorders Center (Boston, MA, USA), High-Impact Cancer Research postgraduate program at Harvard Medical School (Boston, MA, USA), observership at St. Jude Children's Research Hospital (SJCRH) (Memphis, TN, USA), Global Health Delivery Intensive Course at the Harvard School of Public Health (Boston, MA, USA), and countless of seminars, conferences, and short trainings.

During and after every program and training, we were making a new step and organizing a new program, and when looking back, I can state that these programs were life-changing experiences.

Difficulties and Victories

In December 2015, I returned back home. I packed my big baggage to the airport in Boston and then made a few days stop in Orlando for the American Society of Hematology annual meeting, and in a winter day, I landed in Yerevan, my home city.

Why did I return? For two reasons: first, because it is my home, and second, because I was confident that I could make a change. Was it a difficult task? Definitely, it was. Were we able to make a change? Definitely. We were fortunate.

I started working at the Muratsan Hospital of YSMU, at the clinic where I made my first steps in pediatric hematology and oncology, and also lecturing at the oncology department of YSMU.

Of course, there were people who were making obstacles, but altogether, there were always those who were helping to overcome those challenges. One thing I know for sure and I believe in firmly is that if you want something very much, the whole universe will help you to achieve it.

I will try to summarize the achievements we accomplished during the last decade, hoping that these steps could be educational for others.

In 2012, we founded the Armenian Association of Hematology and Oncology (AAHO), the professional union of cancer and blood disorder specialists. Since that time, our team organized and hosted large and small educational and scientific events, which had a significant impact on Armenia. To name few of them are as follows: first American Society of Clinical Oncology (ASCO) Multidisciplinary Cancer Management Course in Armenia, first ASCO joint master class with the European School of Oncology and Pediatric Oncology East and Mediterranean Group second Scientific Congress, first Cancer Survivorship Congress in Armenia, "Conquering Cancer in Armenia with a Smile" International Conference with the MD Anderson Cancer Center and Dana–Farber/Boston Children's Cancer and Blood Disorders Center (DF/BC), first Taiwan–Armenian Medical Congress, International Society on Thrombosis and Haemostasis first Educational Course in Armenia, and many others.

In 2014, our team of physicians founded the City of Smile Foundation (CSF), which later became the largest cancer charity in Armenia and currently is covering the whole diagnosis, treatment, and care for children and young adults from 0 up to 25 years old in Armenia. The foundation also puts much effort in research, capacity building, education, and development. The initial purpose of the foundation was for every cancer patient in Armenia to receive appropriate care regardless of their or their family's financial ability, but later on, the foundation extended its scope. In 2016, with the help from DF/BC, we established the first psychosocial program for cancer patients in Armenia. The program became much larger during the time and now is a well-functioning and important part of our center. In the same year, AAHO signed a memorandum with MD Anderson Cancer Center, which enabled many specialists to get training there and also to start joint research.

In 2016, we started the cancer.am website, analogous to cancer.net, which contains specialist-approved information for the public. The creation of the website was supported by the US Embassy in Armenia and became an important tool for patients, caregivers, and the whole public.

Starting from 2016, with the support from the World Vision, we started training rural pediatricians and GPs in pediatric oncology. For that, we also translated the WHO-PAHO (Pan American Health Organization) guide for the early pediatric cancer diagnosis. Due to this training and the guide, more and more physicians started referring the patients in the early stages.

In 2018, Dr. Danielyan was appointed as a director of the Hematology Center after Prof. R. H. Yeolyan, and this was the catalyst that later in February 2019, we were able to merge all the existing pediatric hematology and oncology units in Armenia and to create a united Pediatric Cancer and Blood Disorders Center of Armenia (PCBDCA), which became part of the Hematology Center, renovated in 2016.

In 2019, Armenia became the first country to join the St. Jude Global Alliance led by the SJCRH. With St. Jude, we have had a long-lasting relation, but this further catalyzed our cooperation (Armenia Becomes First Country to Join St. Jude Global Alliance n.d.).

From the same year, with the support from the Bridge of Health charitable foundation, we started working on the creation of a pediatric cancer registry for Armenia. We went back up to 25 years and started scanning all the medical documentations from every single unit in Armenia, who had a patient with cancer. Later on, we started extracting data from those pdfs and putting in the St. Jude Global Registry. Even though this is a huge amount of work, it will give us very valuable information about the past and the present of pediatric cancer care in Armenia and will help to shape the future.

Another critically important milestone was the establishment of the Department of Pediatric Oncology and Hematology at YSMU in July 2019. We created a 3-year fellowship program for a united "pediatric hematologist–oncologist" specialization and for the first time in the history of Armenia accepted fellows for training in this specialization. For our fellowship program, besides the general requirements, we put special requirements: knowledge of foreign languages (at least English and Russian) and a mandatory requirement of doing a research and publishing a paper in internationally recognized scientific journals. This decision allowed us to accept the best graduates of our medical university. In the first year, we got seven fellows and the next year three fellows, from which one is from Russia. From the first days, fellows got actively involved in the clinical work and started doing research. Already in the first year, 35 abstracts were submitted and accepted at major international congresses. This was a big achievement for a small country like Armenia with such a small field like pediatric hematology–oncology.

In August 2019, we made another important decision on the creation of four multidisciplinary working groups (WGs)—leukemias, lymphomas and SCT (stem cell transplant), solid tumors, neuro-oncology and musculoskeletal tumors. This initiative was supported by the CSF. Each working group has been discussing all cases in a multidisciplinary setting on a weekly basis, involving also foreign experts. In addition, every WG started translating and adapting guidelines for different cancer subtypes. By the end of the first year, we had created already guidelines for 17 cancer subtypes (overall, around 4000 pages

of work), which included a manual for specialists, a manual for primary healthcare providers, and a guide for the patients. This helped us not only produce the guidelines, which was really a unique effort for our country, or have multidisciplinary meetings, but it was a great help for all our staff to update the knowledge and develop their English language skills. We recruited a full-time coordinator for each WG, with medical or public health background. I should state that this step was critical for the success of the project, to have dedicated personnel for coordination. All the members of the WGs were salaried; since the salaries for medical personnel are very low in Armenia, this was also a kind of a salary supplementation and incentive.

Palliative care is an essential part of the cancer care, but it is greatly lacking in our country. In the coming month, we will open the first pediatric cancer palliative care center (hospice) within the PCBDCA, which is a beautiful five-room facility with international standards. It was constructed by the support of CSF. There were many other achievements in recent years, including starting doing high-dose methotrexate for leukemias, brain tumors, and bone sarcomas (5 g/m^2 and more), special training for nurses, active work within international organizations, etc., and with every achievement, of course, there are many difficulties to get there.

Of course, pediatric oncology is a sensitive field. Many people want to help kids with cancer, but when you do some good thing, there are always people, who seem to put hurdles in your way. The phenomenon of small countries is that huge problems can be solved in a minute, but sometimes to solve a tiny problem might take ages and enormous efforts.

Recent years were very productive years, but still there is a lot to do. During a recent interview with a local journalist, I was asked what my dream was, and I responded that no child with cancer would leave Armenia for getting treatment abroad, but just the opposite, children from abroad would come to Armenia to get a high-quality care. Of course, this is a difficult task, but I am sure that day will come. During my not very long career, I understood one thing very clearly that everything is achievable; you just should be persistent and do not pay attention to negative people.

Epilogue

It is Saturday afternoon, March 6, 2021, 26–27 years ago, the same days Dr. Danielyan was sitting in the reception of different business people and authorities, asking for pediatric cancer medications. The majority of those meetings ended with zero results; it was very disappointing. But he was persistent, and the day came. With several kindhearted people, the Hilfe für Armenia Foundation was established in Germany to help children with leukemia living in Armenia. For more than two decades, this foundation became the cornerstone for advancing pediatric leukemia treatment in Armenia, helping to cure more than 1000 children with leukemia.

A long time passed, those children with leukemia now have their own children, but, unfortunately, like in the 1990s, the government is not covering the diagnosis and treatment of these catastrophic diseases. Hence, the physicians need to think not only about medicine but also about making the medicine accessible.

And now I am sitting in the room, in front of the laptop screen and sending emails to the people around the world. I do not know most of them. I found their names in the list of philanthropists of Armenian and foreign organizations, churches, and community organizations. The majority of them do not have a publicly available email, and it usually takes time and efforts to get any contact from them. And in the early morning, when they wake up, they are going to open their mailbox and find an email entitled "Help request for pediatric cancer patients in Armenia" from a person from Armenia, about whom they have never heard. Most of them will not answer to this spam-like email; few of them will reply but will regret about not being able to help, and only one or two answers from tens (sometimes hundred) of emails will be positive! But those positive emails definitely will come; one just needs to be persistent and not give up. And those 1–2 emails will be the catalysts of change!

References

Armenia Becomes First Country to Join St. Jude Global Alliance (n.d.) https://www.commercialappeal.com/story/news/2019/04/12/st-jude-childrens-research-hospital-st-jude-global-alliance-armenia-childhood-cancer/3445747002/. Accessed 10 March 2021

Childhood Cancer (n.d.) https://www.who.int/news-room/fact-sheets/detail/cancer-in-children. Accessed 10 March 2021

Danielyan S (2009) Treatment achievements, challenges and perspectives of childhood leukemias in Armenia. New Armen Med J 3(3):91

Danielyan S, Iskanyan S (2004) Treatment outcomes of childhood leukemias after the implementation of BFM program. Med Armen 44(1):86–87

Danielyan S, Vagharshakyan L, Zakharyan A, Iskanyan S, Arakelyan S (2020) Increasing the effectiveness of treatment among children with leukemia in the Republic of Armenia. Eurasian J Oncol Clin Med 1:39–42

Hovhannisyan S, Papyan R, Sargsyan L, Danielyan S, Vagharshakyan L, Avagyan A et al (2020) Pediatric cancer care in Armenia: the results of a qualitative analysis. J Clin Oncol 38(Suppl):abstract e19002

Papyan R (2018) The state of pediatric oncology in Armenia: challenges and achievements. In: American Society of Pediatric Hematology and Oncology Annual Meeting. N. 648

Steinherz P (1987) Acute lymphoblastic leukemia of childhood. Hematol Oncol Clin North Am 1(4):549–566

Tamamyan G (2020) Pediatric oncology in the Republic of Armenia: developments in recent years. Med. Sci Educ:68–72

Wikipedia: Armenia (n.d.) https://en.wikipedia.org/wiki/Armenia. Accessed 10 March 2021

Quality Oncology Practice Improvement (QOPI) in Brazil: A Successful Knowledge Transfer Under the Auspices of the American Society of Clinical Oncology (ASCO)

Rodrigo Cunha Guimaraes, Pedro Ribeiro Santos, and Bruno Lemos Ferrari

Introduction

Although it is supposed that physicians' knowledge increases over time, there are some data that suggest the quality of care delivered to the patients by a physician decreases over the years of clinical practice (Choudhry et al. 2005). Physicians may derive benefit from quality programs to keep delivering a high-quality care to their patients (Hockey and Marshall 2009). For instance, quality programs encourage physicians to take part in continuing medical education, as well as to work on other scientific activities.

Outpatient oncology practices are complex organizations. They are composed of a multidisciplinary team involved in the therapeutic management of cancer patients, including medical specialists, nurses, pharmacists, social workers, psychologists, nutritionists, dentists, and administrative staff. Clear communication among professionals providing care to a group of patients is essential to prevent errors and maximize treatment results (Pfeiffer et al. 2018). Goals, efficiency measures, and compliance norms should be registered to allow assessment of the results. Quality programs have been developed to warrant a thorough assessment of the patient in the oncology practice, as well as to offer training in how to properly perform patient identification, drug preparation, drug dispensing, and drug administration.

QOPI

The Quality Oncology Practice Initiative (QOPI®) is a quality program developed by the American Society of Clinical Oncology (ASCO®). The QOPI pilot program was launched in 2002 and completed in 2005. As of 2006, QOPI program has been opened for applications, since the oncology practices were from the United States and had medical oncologists who were ASCO members (McNiff 2006). As of 2016, ASCO has broadened QOPI applications, extending to practices from other countries (Blayney et al. 2020).

The program has been designed for outpatient oncology practices with the aim of improving

R. C. Guimaraes (✉) · P. R. Santos
Department of Medical Oncology, Oncocentro de Minas Gerais, Belo Horizonte, Minas Gerais, Brazil
e-mail: rodrigo.guimaraes@medicos.oncoclinicas.com; pedro.santos@medicos.oncoclinicas.com

B. L. Ferrari
Department of Medical Oncology, Oncocentro de Minas Gerais, Belo Horizonte, Minas Gerais, Brazil

Oncoclinicas Group, São Paulo, SP, Brazil
e-mail: bruno.ferrari@oncoclinicas.com

U. Schmidt-Strassburger (ed.), *Improving Oncology Worldwide*, Sustainable Development Goals Series,
https://doi.org/10.1007/978-3-030-96053-7_17

patient quality care, as well as developing a culture of self-examination. In order to participate in the QOPI, the practice must have a professional with an active ASCO membership.

Through the QOPI portal, registered practices can report more than 150 quality measures in different areas, receiving detailed performance reports, with the possibility of benchmarking with all participating practices. In addition, clinics that achieve a minimum of 75% compliance with these measures can apply for the QOPI certification program (QCP™).

QCP

The QOPI Certification Program (QCP) is an accreditation that recognizes high-quality care for outpatient hematology-oncology practices. The QCP has standards that the clinic must follow in order to receive certification (Neuss et al. 2016).

They are divided into the following four domains:

Creating a Safe Environment— Staffing and General Policy

At least eight elements should be documented in the medical chart before a new chemotherapeutic regimen such as the following:

1. Pathologic confirmation or verification of initial diagnosis.
2. Initial cancer stage or current status.
3. Complete medical history and physical examination, including pregnancy status.
4. Presence or absence of allergies and history of hypersensitivity reactions.
5. Assessment of the patient's and/or caregiver's comprehension of information regarding the disease and treatment plan.
6. Initial psychosocial assessment, with action taken when indicated.
7. The chemotherapeutic treatment plan, including, at a minimum, the patient diagnosis, drugs, doses, duration of treatment, and goals of therapy.

8. Planned frequency of office visits and patient monitoring that is appropriate for the individual chemotherapy agents.

Treatment Planning, Patient Consent, and Education

The oncology practice should have a policy that documents a standardized process for obtaining and documenting chemotherapy consent. Patient or caregiver should be informed about goals of the treatment, if there is intention to cure, prolong life, or reduce symptoms, as well as potential long-term and short-term adverse effects of therapy, including infertility risks for appropriate patients.

Ordering, Preparing, Dispensing, and Administering Chemotherapy

The oncology practice should have a policy for chemotherapy orders that ensure that verbal orders are not allowed except to hold or stop chemotherapy administration. New orders or modifications are documented in the medical record. Chemotherapy orders include at least the following elements:

- The patient's name.
- Patient identifier.
- Date.
- Regimen or protocol name and number.
- Cycle number and day, when applicable.
- All medications within the order set that are listed by using full generic names.
- Drug dose which is written following standards for abbreviations, trailing zeros, and leading zeros.

The oncology practice pharmacy should have a policy regarding the safe storage of chemotherapy, including separation of look-alike products and investigational agents available in multiple strengths.

Before administration of each chemotherapy cycle, the practitioner who is administering the chemotherapy confirms the treatment with the patient, including, at a minimum, the name of the drug, infusion time, and infusion-related symptoms to report. At least two individuals verify the patient identification by using at least two identifiers, in the presence of the patient. The management of extravasation should be aligned with current literature and guidelines.

Following Up The Patient After Chemotherapy Administration, Including Adherence, Toxicity, and Complications

The oncology practice should use standard disease-specific processes to monitor treatment response and has a policy that determines the appropriate time interval for regimen-specific tests, based on evidence and national guidelines when available. Cumulative doses of chemotherapy are tracked for agents associated with cumulative toxicity.

The assessment is made on a one-day on-site survey when the ASCO team assesses whether all standards are met. If 100% of the standards are met, the practice is certified.

The Oncocentro Experience

The Oncoclinicas Group, founded in 2010, is one of the largest networks of oncology, hematology, and radiation oncology in Latin America. The area of operation of the Oncoclinicas Group covers 11 of the main Brazilian states. Currently, there are 68 facilities which have medical specialists in the fields of medical oncology, radiation oncology, hematology, bone marrow transplantation, integrative medicine, and the most advanced clinical care.

Initially, the group selected 6 practices to apply for the QOPI quality certification (QCP). One of them was Oncocentro, located in the city of Belo Horizonte in the state of Minas Gerais.

The Oncocentro process started in May 2019 with the selection of a coordinator physician with an active ASCO membership, the so-called QOPI champion. From then on, a team composed of a nurse and a pharmacist was formed in association with the physician. In the first stage, the clinic registered to the QOPI and started collecting data from medical charts in the minimum required modules, which were symptoms and toxicity, breast cancer, lung cancer, colorectal cancer, and gynecological cancer. Based on the number of the medical oncologists in the practice, it was required a minimum of 80 medical charts in each of these modules.

The data collection process took approximately 6 months, and at the end, 89.91% of compliance had been obtained, and therefore, the clinic was considered able to apply for the QCP.

In parallel with data collection, the entire clinical staff of the practice was mobilized to meet the QCP standards. Many of the standards had already been implemented due to other quality processes previously experienced by the clinic. At that time, Oncocentro had already been certified by the Joint Commission International (JCI) and by the National Accreditation Organization (NAO). Several quality and safety standards had already been met, but adjustments had to be made in some policies to better meet the QCP standards.

Along with Oncocentro, Oncoclinicas Group staff and leaders of the five other practices held weekly meetings to share experiences and obstacles. Teamwork and collaboration among practices gave meaningful support during the preparation for the QCP. In addition, the ASCO International Quality Team offered an essential guidance throughout the process, being always available and very professional.

In February 2020, Oncocentro was visited by ASCO International Quality team for the on-site survey. During the visit, all standards were evaluated, including the process of ordering, preparing, dispensing, and administering chemotherapy.

After the visit, it was a pleasure to learn that Oncocentro had met 100% compliance with the standards of QCP, thereby becoming a QOPI-certified practice. All of the other five practices of Oncoclinicas Group were also certified.

For Oncocentro, participating in QOPI and being certified by the QCP was paramount. In addition to confirming the clinic is committed to the best practices in oncology, the seal states that it has achieved high standard safety and quality parameters in several areas of activity, including training and qualification of the team, strict control of order, preparation and administration of chemotherapy, and appropriate follow-up of patients after treatment.

References

Blayney DW, Albdelhafeez N, Jazieh AR, Pinto CF, Udrea A, Roach A, Das D, Grubbs S, Hamm J, Jahanzeb M, Kamal AH, Kelly RJ, Martin SE, O'Mahony D, Birch W, Bowman R, Crist STS, Evers A, Gilmore T, Klein M, Siegel R (2020) International perspective on the pursuit of quality in cancer care: global application of QOPI and QOPI certification. JCO Glob Oncol 6:697–703. https://doi.org/10.1200/GO.20.00048. PMID: 32374622; PMCID: PMC7268902

Choudhry NK, Fletcher RH, Soumerai SB (2005) Systematic review: the relationship between clinical experience and quality of health care. Ann Intern Med 142(4):260–273. https://doi.org/10.7326/0003-4819-142-4-200502150-00008

Hockey PM, Marshall MN (2009) Doctors and quality improvement. J R Soc Med 102(5):173–176. https://doi.org/10.1258/jrsm.2009.090065. PMID: 19417048; PMCID: PMC2677433

McNiff K (2006) The quality oncology practice initiative: assessing and improving care within the medical oncology practice. J Oncol Pract 2(1):26–30. https://doi.org/10.1200/JOP.2006.2.1.26. PMID: 20871730; PMCID: PMC2794634

Neuss MN, Gilmore TR, Belderson KM, Billet AL, Kalchik TC, Harvey BE, Hendricks C, LeFebvre KB, Mangu PB, McNiff K, Olsen M, Schulmeister L, Gehr AV, Polovich M (2016) Updated American Society of Clinical Oncology/Oncology Nursing Society. Chemotherapy Administration Safety Standards, Including Standards for Pediatric Oncology. J Oncol Pract 12(12):1262–1271. https://doi.org/10.1200/JOP.2016.0107905

Pfeiffer Y, Gut SS, Schwappach DLB (2018) Medication safety in oncology care: mapping checking procedures from prescription to Administration of Chemotherapy. J Oncol Pract 14(4):e201–e210. https://doi.org/10.1200/JOP.2017.026427. Epub 2018 Feb 26

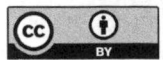

Challenges in Running a Comprehensive Cancer Center

Thomas Seufferlein

Introduction

The concept of a Comprehensive Cancer Center was first develpoed in France French Comprehensive Cancer Centers (2021). As we practice it here in Germany it is rather similar to the concept that has been established in the USA National Comprehensive Cancer Network: NCCN (2021). Comprehensive Cancer Centers are expected to initiate and conduct early phase, innovative clinical trials and to actively participate in trials of the National Cancer Institute (NCI) of the USA and in turn receive funding from the NCI. They must show activities in outreach and education both for health-care professionals and the public and demonstrate expertise in laboratory, clinical, epidemiological, and health-care research National Comprehensive Cancer Network: NCCN (2021). This concept has been adapted by other countries including Germany. Here, with a different structure of health-care delivery, CCCs exhibit close similarities but also slight differences to the structure in the USA (Das Netzwerk der Onkologischen Spitzenzentren (2021); Deutsche Krebshilfe: Onkologische Spitzenzentren (2021)). Running a CCC is challenging at several levels that are outlined in this paper.

T. Seufferlein (✉)
Department of Internal Medicine I, Ulm University Hospital and Ulm Comprehensive Cancer Center CCCU, Ulm, Germany
e-mail: thomas.seufferlein@uniklinik-ulm.de

The core features of a CCC in Germany are shown in Fig. 1.

Multidisciplinary Tumor Boards

The multidisciplinary tumor boards are at the heart of the clinical management of patients in a CCC. The boards meet regularly (at least weekly), and the participation of all specialties involved in the treatment of a certain tumor entity is mandatory. For example, for gastrointestinal (GI) cancer, the tumor board comprises visceral surgery, GI oncology, gastroenterology, pathology, radiology, radiation therapy, and nuclear medicine. The board discusses all patients newly diagnosed with a GI cancer, relapsed patients, patients with a change of strategy (e.g., secondary resection of liver metastases after chemotherapy), and patients having received procedures (e.g., TACE or SIRT). This means that patients are usually presented several times in the tumor board during their continuum of care. This is challenging particularly for cross-sectional specialties like pathology and radiology that have to attend multiple tumor boards, which is time-consuming both for preparing and attending and demanding for a specialty since the requirement for participating in a tumor board is consultant level. Qualification is important because decisions taken by the board should not be overturned by a single specialty unless for good reasons. Participation of the respective spe-

U. Schmidt-Strassburger (ed.), *Improving Oncology Worldwide*, Sustainable Development Goals Series,
https://doi.org/10.1007/978-3-030-96053-7_18

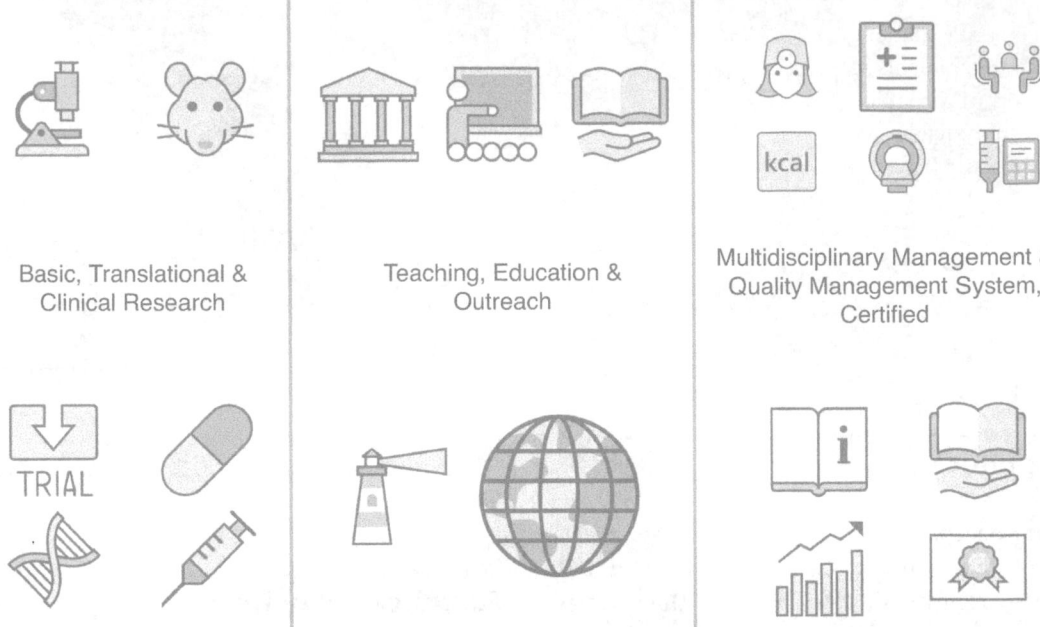

Fig. 1 Core features of a CCC in Germany. Left—Strong and comprehensive research and clinical trial program. Center—Supraregional education and teaching in oncology and outreach program. Right—Established structure in the multidisciplinary management of cancer care in all specialties including psychooncology, nutritionists, patient self-help groups, and social work follows all current guidelines in oncology and has an established quality management system, certified by an established certification system

cialties as well as adherence to the criteria defined above and the tumor board decisions are regularly monitored. Unfortunately, there is no funding structure allowing to compensate for the additional time it takes to prepare and carry out the tumor boards.

IT Infrastructure

IT infrastructure of a CCC comprises various aspects: electronic patients' records, a tumor board management system, a trial management system, and a cancer registry software ideally all interlinked in order to facilitate documentation and avoid repetitive entries into different databases.

This can be exemplified with a tumor board management system. Using an advanced and well-linked tumor board management system has several key advantages: data entry is only once and can be taken over by all documentation systems during the continuum of treatment of a given patient. With the introduction of mandatory fields in the documentation system, one can make sure that all the necessary information to take a sensible decision in the tumor board is actually available. This enables also better second-opinion decisions particularly when the treating physician is not able to present the patient's case in person in the tumor board. Such a system can also list clinical trials running at the site the patient may be eligible for and should enable an on the spot, transparent documentation of the tumor board decision.

A clinical trial management system is also extremely useful when it is fully integrated into the hospital's patient management system. First of all, it provides an easy overview on all trials running at the center and on all patients recruited into a specific trial. Furthermore, it can immediately indicate in an emergency that a certain patient participates in a clinical trial when they are seen at the hospital's A&E department. Upon admission of a patient, the physicians can see whether the patient is on a trial, the kind of treatment the patients receive, learn the potential side effects of the study medication, get in touch with the study team, and choose an appropriate treatment if the patient's condition has been judged as study treatment related. Ideally both the tumor management system and the clinical trial management system are also closely linked to the tumor documentation system. We developed our own system called CREDOS for Cancer Retrieval Evaluation and Documentation System that is linked to all other systems described above and fulfills all the statutory criteria for the official tumor documentation. It also enables the documentation of all items required for the certification of our CCC as an "Oncology Center" by the German Cancer Society. The major advantage of having a proprietary system is that it allows customization to the ever-changing needs in cancer documentation, for example, with the upcoming requirement of documenting data from NGS (next-generation sequencing) used for molecular characterization of a tumor and personalized treatment of patients. Having said all of that, setting up and maintaining such an IT infrastructure which goes beyond the standard setting of a university hospital requires resources that are not included in the regular funding schemes.

Structuring Patient Care

Ideally multidisciplinarity in a CCC is not only practiced at the level of the tumor boards, SOPs (standard operating procedures), and clinical trials but also at the level of direct patient care. This includes interdisciplinary management teams, for example, in an outpatient clinic for GI cancers that is run by a GI oncologist and a surgeon with an additional radiotherapist or other specialties (e.g., nuclear medicine) if need be. Here the patient gets a comprehensive assessment and treatment concept from all parties involved in the management of their disease, and all questions and issues can be addressed appropriately. This type of clinic is also very useful for patients seeking a second opinion on their case.

Clinical Trial Center

Since CCCs are in charge of both delivery of care and research, they are the ideal structures to run innovative high-level clinical trials, particularly investigator-initiated trials and phase I/phase II including first in human trials. To this end, they need well-structured clinical trial centers that accompany the whole process from writing the protocol up to negotiating contracts and initiating and monitoring multicenter trials. This does not only require trained study nurses and physicians, a quality management, and an education infrastructure, for example, for GCP courses, but also an appropriate IT infrastructure. The number of patients included into clinical trials in each tumor entity is monitored. In solid tumors, at least 10% of the patients seen at the center should be included into a clinical trial.

Research Infrastructure

Additional, but important, features of a CCC are access to a modern research infrastructure including genomics, proteomics, and bioinformatics. A CCC needs an established and well-maintained biobank. This comprises ideally not only paraffin embedded but also the fresh frozen normal and tumor tissue, liquid biobanks (e.g., for analysis of ctDNA, circulating tumor cells, or hematological tumors), a stool biobank (for microbiota analyses), and various other analytes including urine and ascites.

Well-annotated biobanks are a paramount prerequisite for personalizing tumor therapy and establishing novel prognostic and predictive biomarkers for various oncological treatments. They also feed into collaborative research centers, research training groups, and other basic and translational research units at a respective site.

Care Over and Above Medical Treatment

In recent years, it has become more and more evident that apart from excellent medical care, cancer patients also need structured help in many other areas to cope with their disease. This is particularly important with prolonged periods of treatment and consequently more side effects of the treatment and a higher burden for patients. Thus, psychooncology care is an important feature of a CCC and reaches from the cancer diagnosis to the time a patient has survived cancer but still suffers from treatment-related side effects or psychological constraints. In this context, also social work is important to avoid financial difficulties and support the well-being of the patient. Also, other aspects need to be taken into account in a CCC: physical exercise is an important measure to improve outcome of a particular treatment, accelerate rehabilitation, and improve quality of life during chemotherapy and also for secondary and tertiary prevention of cancer. Thus, structured programs for exercise therapy are another part of the comprehensive cancer care in a CCC. Last but not least, nutrition is also important in cancer care, and oncological nutritional counseling is another important component of a comprehensive cancer care package in a CCC. All these structures require less investment but appropriate and sustainable staffing to be successful thereby creating a challenge for the financial resources of a CCC.

Quality Management

Given all the requirements stated above, it is clear that a CCC needs a clearly defined quality management system. Regular quality circles aim at recognizing, discussing, and detecting problems and challenges as early as possible. These circles take place every 3 months. All parties involved in the tumor boards are invited to these circles. The circles are logged, and the decisions taken are important components for the further development of the center.

Regular mortality and morbidity (M&M) conferences are another, very important hallmark of the quality management. They also take place four times a year and review particular treatment histories and deaths. The M&M conferences aim at deriving concrete measures to improve the quality and safety of patient care at the center and to avoid potential mistakes in the future as much as possible.

Quality management also encompasses regular surveys of referring physicians and patients regarding satisfaction with the services provided by the center. The evaluation of these surveys is also the basis for the action plan of the Comprehensive Cancer Center Ulm (CCCU) (2021) since reducing cancer-related morbidity and mortality is the overarching goal of these centers.

Structuring the Clinical Work

A CCC shall define how it operates and has to define multidisciplinary standard operating procedures for all tumor entities treated but also for all supportive measures taken by the CCC. They shall be consented by all participating parties and must be updated regularly. In case of the CCCU, these are 53 SOPs covering different tumor entities and 39 SOPs for supportive treatment. This is a time-consuming and laborious task, since these guidelines are based on international and national guidelines, double-checked for subject-specific demands of all disciplines involved, and innovation must be covered in word and deed. All SOPs must also be consented by the cooperating partners, and their input shall be taken into account to ensure that the whole catchment area of the CCC follows the same SOPs.

Outreach Activities

A very important part of the activities of a CCC is outreach. The goal is to provide state-of-the-art care in oncology not only at the center itself but in the whole catchment area of the CCC. For this purpose, a CCC will set up a network of cooperating centers (in case of Germany either hospitals or private practices). Within this network, regular education and training activities as well as information on novel clinical trials the peripheral centers take place. These activities result in referring patients for inclusion or becoming recruiting centers themselves. There is not only education for physicians with seminars and lectures but also structured activities such as a master's program in advanced oncology and joint postgraduate education with collaboration partners. Ideally, there are also structured training programs for oncology nurses. An important part of the outreach program is the interaction with patient self-help groups and educating patients and their relatives and learning their needs. For this purpose, the CCC organizes regular educational events together with patient self-help groups on various topics covering not only medical issues but also psychooncology and social support for cancer patients and their families.

Getting Funded

In contrast to the USA with a National Cancer Institute that provides funding for CCCs, there is no such structure in Germany. Thus, the CCCs receive only the regular funding for cancer documentation, but there is no overhead paid by the statutory health insurances or the federal and regional authorities to support the complex CCC structure outlined above. The German Cancer Aid, a charity dedicated to support research and treatment of cancer in all aspects, has launched a program funding CCCs when they fulfill certain criteria that are evaluated regularly by an international expert panel in audits. This provides funding for some aspects of a CCC but does not fully support the structure and is not an overarching structure providing enrollment into clinical trials. There is therefore a high level of commitment by all parties contributing to the CCC supporting the structure with staff as well as resources from their own departments as well as raising money from third parties.

Conclusion

In conclusion, running a comprehensive cancer center is a continuous process and development that is absolutely worthwhile to further improve treatment for cancer patients in all aspects. It takes time to completely implement all the components of a CCC. Working in multidisciplinary teams and combining clinical excellence with research is the philosophy of a CCC and broadens the clinical horizon. A major challenge in running a CCC is funding, but with commitment and enthusiasm, a CCC can achieve excellent results in a good multidisciplinary atmosphere promoting basic, translational, and clinical science. And with all of that, it helps our patients and their families.

References

Comprehensive Cancer Center Ulm (2021) https://www.uniklinik-ulm.de/comprehensive-cancer-center-ulm-cccu.html. Accessed 10 March 2021

Das Netzwerk der Onkologischen Spitzenzentren (2021) http://www.ccc-netzwerk.de. Accessed 10 March 2021

Deutsche Krebshilfe: Onkologische Spitzenzentren (2021) https://www.krebshilfe.de/helfen/rat-hilfe/onkologische-spitzenzentren. Accessed 10 March 2021

French Comprehensive Cancer Centers (2021) http://www.unicancer.fr/en/patients/french-comprehensive-cancer-centers Accessed 10 March 2021

National Comprehensive Cancer Network: NCCN (2021) https://www.nccn.org. Accessed 10 March 2021

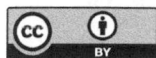

Index

CPSIA information can be obtained
at www.ICGtesting.com
Printed in the USA
LVHW060109230622
721928LV00008B/484